Developmental Speech-Language Training through Music for Children with Autism Spectrum Disorders

of related interest

Music Therapy, Sensory Integration and the Autistic Child
Dorita S. Berger
Foreword by Donna Williams
ISBN 978 1 84310 700 2

Music Therapy in Schools
21st Century Trends and Developments
Edited by Jo Tomlinson, Philippa Derrington and Amelia Oldfield
ISBN 978 1 84905 000 5

Music Therapy with Children and their Families
Edited by Amelia Oldfield and Claire Flower
Foreword by Vince Hesketh
ISBN 978 1 84310 581 7

Let's All Listen
Songs for Group Work in Settings that Include Students with Learning Difficulties and Autism
Pat Lloyd
Foreword by Adam Ockelford
ISBN 978 1 84310 583 1

Music for Special Kids
Musical Activities, Songs, Instruments and Resources
Pamela Ott
ISBN 978 1 84905 858 2

Developmental Speech-Language Training through Music for Children with Autism Spectrum Disorders

Theory and Clinical Application

Hayoung A. Lim, PhD, MT-BC
Foreword by Karen E. Miller

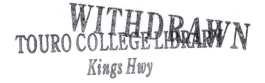
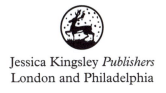

Jessica Kingsley *Publishers*
London and Philadelphia

KH

First published in 2012
by Jessica Kingsley Publishers
116 Pentonville Road
London N1 9JB, UK
and
400 Market Street, Suite 400
Philadelphia, PA 19106, USA

www.jkp.com

Library of Congress Cataloging in Publication Data
Lim, Hayoung A.
 Developmental speech-language training through music for children with
autism spectrum disorders : theory and clinical application / Hayoung A. Lim ;
foreword by Karen Miller.
     p. cm.
 Includes bibliographical references and index.
 ISBN 978-1-84905-849-0 (alk. paper)
 1. Music therapy. 2. Speech therapy. 3. Autism spectrum disorders in
children. 4. Children with autism spectrum disorders--Rehabilitation. I.
Title.
 ML3920.L694 2012
 615.8'51540835--dc22
                    2011010173

British Library Cataloguing in Publication Data
A CIP catalogue record for this book is available from the British Library

ISBN 978 1 84905 849 0

Printed and bound in Great Britain

11/17/16

*I dedicate this book to my husband Timothy
and my son Yeru*

*To Timothy, who has provided me unlimited
encouragement and love*

*To Yeru, who has taught me the effect of
singing on one's development in the most
powerful, yet beautiful, way*

Contents

Part II Developmental Speech and Language Training through Music for Children with ASD: Clinical Implications and Practice

Foreword

Parents, caregivers, researchers, and other observers have long reported notable responses to music by individuals diagnosed with autism spectrum disorders (ASD). Responses range from increased attention to musical stimuli and a strong motivation for music-related activity to significant gains in non-musical, functional development through the therapeutic uses of music. While investigation in this area is ongoing, the growing research base continues to support the notion that music can be used as an effective therapeutic tool for many diagnosed with ASD.

Clinically based research studies have shown benefit for quite some time, while more recent research demonstrates increased focus on the scientific rationale for functional outcomes. One area of particular interest has been the impact of music on speech and language development and the neurological mechanisms responsible for functional gains. In this book, Dr Lim combines her passions for research, education, and clinical practice in the development of an important work: this work is characterized by a careful and thorough review of current literature, including a review of her own research studies and clinical experiences, and a systematic, detailed explanation of suggested treatment protocols. The result is an in-depth study of research-based music therapy techniques used to improve speech and language skills of young children with ASD.

Any sound therapeutic profession must be built on a foundation of research, theory, and practical application. Music therapy is no exception. In this highly useful book, Dr Lim clearly provides an explanation of all three as they relate to the speech and language of children with ASD. She also gives a thorough introduction to the applied behavior analysis (ABA) approach to speech and language development in autism and clearly articulates the compatibility between developmental speech and language training through music (DSLM) and the widely utilized ABA approach. The book is both theoretical and highly practical, and both theory and method are supported by an extensive review of the current research literature.

The uniqueness and importance of the work go hand in hand. It is unique in its focus on a specific domain of development (speech and language) and a particular diagnostic category (ASD), whereas most current manuals within the field of music therapy address a broader spectrum of domains and/or diagnoses. The result of Dr Lim's focus is an in-depth exploration of the topic from research, theoretical, and practical vantage points.

As the field of music therapy continues to broaden and expand, it is increasingly important for therapists and researchers alike to deepen their knowledge of particular treatments and their clinical and scientific rationales, and then to explore the possibility of transferring ideas, techniques, and protocols to other areas of research and treatment as indicated. This book offers the opportunity to move forward in that process by gaining a more thorough understanding of music's potential to improve the speech and language of young children with ASD.

Karen E. Miller, MM, MT-BC
Director of Music Therapy
Sam Houston State University

Preface

It is a true honor to write a book about my own experiences as a music therapy clinician and researcher for children with autism. The number of American children diagnosed with autism has skyrocketed in the past decades, causing widespread concern and confusion. Since Leo Kanner's first description of infantile autism in 1943, the occurrence has climbed to an alarming 1 in 150 people across the United States. Autism seems to be on the rise, and autism spectrum disorders (ASD) affect between two and six children out of every thousand in the United States. Currently there is no cure for autism, though with early intervention and treatment, the diverse symptoms related to autism can be greatly improved. Speech and language impairment has been regarded as one of the most significant deficits in autism. Most parents of children with autism first begin to be concerned that something is not quite right in their child's development when early delay or regression occurs in the development of language. The parents of children with autism have identified speech and language impairment as one of the most significant stresses they experience with their children in the preschool and school years. A deficit in the communicative use of language is a defining feature of autism, and it directly reflects the core developmental difficulties of children with autism. Effective intervention therefore is needed in the development of social communication including speech and language.

In 2009, the president of the American Music Therapy Association (AMTA) announced that ASD is the clinical population which gets most priority in music therapy services and research. Before coming to Sam Houston State University as director of graduate studies in music therapy, I worked in children's health and education management in Miami, Florida, as the autism-specialized music therapist. Most of my clients were preschoolers, and they received individual and group music therapy sessions emphasizing speech and language training every week.

My typical music therapy session began with a song called "Music time," which goes like this:

> This is music time, this is a fun time. Everybody can sing and play, everybody is happy.

There was a girl, Vicky, who was four and had been diagnosed with ASD. When I met Vicky for music therapy assessment, she was not able to speak any functional vocabulary words. So, the most critical goal for her music therapy was to increase speech and language. From the first session, I could tell Vicky liked music, particularly singing. She made good eye contact with me whenever I sang, and had a good rhythmic sense. She could copy most of my beats on the drum or rhythm sticks. Her favorite instrument was the egg shaker, and she enjoyed playing the egg shakers as an accompaniment to my singing.

In the fifth session with Vicky, I started our music therapy session with the "Music time" song like this:

> This is music time, this is a fun time. Vicky can sing and play, Vicky is _____.

I made a little pause right before the end of the song. And Vicky said "Happy" with a very clear and loud voice. I called in Vicky's mom and sang the song again. Vicky shouted "Happy" again in front of her mom. Can you imagine Vicky's mom's reaction after hearing her daughter's very first word "Happy"? Of course, she cried for a long time. Vicky continued filling in the blanks for most of the songs I composed for her music therapy sessions. She started to appropriately use those words outside of her music therapy sessions as well.

While working with children with autism in Miami, I was also pursuing a PhD degree at the University of Miami and gathering resources for my dissertation. From my own clinical experience with many children with ASD, I wanted to prove the effectiveness of my music therapy protocol on speech production in children with autism. Vicky was not the only child who had developed speech and language through singing and various musical experiences. Therefore, the direction for my PhD dissertation research was established. The purpose of the research study was to explore how the perception of music impacts the perception and production of speech, and to examine the effect of music as part of developmental speech and language training for children with ASD. The study compared the effect of speech training and music training on the verbal production of preschoolers with ASD.

I composed six songs for the study (see Appendix A) and the songs included thirty-six target words or two-word phrases (see Appendix B). Each song lyric included six target words/phrases, and each lyric line ended with a target word/phrase and an appropriate musical cadence. Each song was composed in a distinctly different style with a different key, tempo, and meter. In particular, the arrangement of musical elements within the songs was developmentally appropriate for preschoolers; all six songs included melodies within a limited pitch range, close intervals, and repetitive melody lines. Pronunciation of the target words/phrases was emphasized by the rhythmic and harmonic structure as needed to preserve prosody and speech rhythm. In addition, the musical stimuli in my study and music therapy protocols were organized by Gestalt laws of perception including simplicity, similarity, proximity, common direction (i.e. good continuation), and completion (see Chapter 3). Through my clinical experiences, I could predict that the inherent musical structures and organized musical patterns in the six songs would provide a perceptual Gestalt to facilitate processing of both musical and speech information. Each phrase or segment of the six songs was composed with a melody combined with a simple rhythmic figure which was repeated in each song. As a result of the repetition and similarity in musical patterns, the young listeners might have developed familiarity with the music stimuli which could support learning new vocabulary words.

In the study, one group of children received music training. In the music training, a female music student sang the six songs and showed the pictures for the target words/phrases. Another group of children received speech training. The same texts and pictures for the six songs used in the music training were used for the six stories in the speech training session. The third group of children was assigned to the no-training condition. Children's verbal production including semantics, phonology, pragmatics, and prosody was measured by the verbal production evaluation scale (VPES) that I designed (see Appendix C). Results showed that participants in both music and speech training significantly increased their scores on the VPES from the pre-test to the post-test. Both music and speech training were effective for enhancing speech production in children with autism. Children who received music training gained higher scores than participants who received speech training; however, the difference between music and speech was not very significant. Music training was as effective as speech training for improving speech production, and children with autism perceived and produced the linguistic information from music as they do from speech.

When I classified the participants into high functioning children and low functioning children, I found that high functioning children with ASD improved their speech from either music or speech training; however, low functioning participants showed a greater improvement after the music training than the speech training. Low functioning children with autism responded more attentively to music and perceive important linguistic information embedded in those songs. As a result, they could acquire and produce functional vocabulary words.

The scientific mechanisms of my study was that the verbal information in both music and speech conditions utilized a common Gestalt law of perception—the law of good continuation, which involves perceptual completion. Let me give you an example. If I sing the very first part (e.g. "You are my _____") of the well-known song "You are my sunshine," the majority of the listeners will fill out sunshine by singing the word in a second. They cannot suppress singing the missing or uncompleted part of one well-known phrase of "You are my sunshine." Once we have perceived a pattern of stimuli like "You are my sunshine", when the pattern is presented again in an incomplete form or structure, we naturally want to perceive it as a completed one, and finally complete the pattern by filling out or producing the missing part of the pattern. The great thing is that children with autism also appear to have an intact ability to perceive musical and speech patterns and produce the patterns in the same way we do. They utilize the same principle of Gestalt pattern perceptual organization to perceive and produce speech. That's why, in my study, the target words/phrases in both the music and speech stimuli were placed at the end of each phrase, which allowed the children to anticipate the location and time of the target words/phrases to be produced.

Interestingly, I found that children with ASD who received the music training produced more target words/phrases that were conveyed in the musical patterns than the children who received the speech training. This finding suggests that music provides more predictable temporal patterns than speech does, making it easier to be perceived by children with ASD. These findings suggest that the pattern organization facilitated the perception of target words/phrases, and children with ASD can perceive and produce target words/phrases that are embedded in simple and repetitive combinations of musical patterns that are symmetrical and parallel in form organized with the Gestalt laws of perception. Some of the unique structural characteristics in the music were not found in the speech. For example, the law of proximity and the law of similarity were not utilized in the speech stimuli as much as in the music. Participants who received the speech training, therefore, might not have experienced the same level of anticipation and familiarity for the speech patterns in the stories as in the musical pattern in the songs. Collectively, children with ASD respond to music attentively and perceive a good amount of information conveyed in musical stimuli which are organized by principles of pattern perception, and they produce the functional speech as a result. The superior performance on speech production as well as enhanced attention and anticipation in the participants who received music training is explained by the characteristics and inherent structure of music stimuli and their response to the music.

The findings of my study indicate that children with ASD are able to perceive linguistic information, including semantics, phonology, pragmatics, and prosody, which are organized by musical patterns. Children with ASD are able to transform the information perceived as musical patterns into speech patterns. In my study, children with ASD who received music training perceived musical stimuli from six songs; however, they produced speech as the outcome, which is a non-musical, functional behavior. In the post-test, I spoke to all of the children and showed the picture for the target words/phrases. They spoke the target words/phrases back to me. I did not sing and they did not sing back to me. Children with ASD have a certain degree of intact perceptual association between music and speech, and they are able to produce the linguistic information in speech patterns, which was transformed from the musical stimuli.

Structurally and functionally organized music experiences may enhance speech production and vocabulary acquisition in children with ASD. The results of my research study indicate that children with ASD can improve their speech production after receiving a short-term (three days) speech and language intervention. This finding agrees with previous research indicating that, although children with ASD clearly have language impairments, they may also have an intact ability to perceive and produce speech sounds, and may be able to develop some level of functional speech. Music is an effective tool for improving acquisition of functional vocabulary words and speech production in children with ASD. My research suggests that developmental speech and language training through music (DSLM) is as effective as speech training for improving speech production in children with ASD. Improved speech and use of language might help children with ASD to develop communication skills, and experience more conversations and active interactions with others.

Music has been commonly used in autism treatment as a behavioral and developmental method. Music is interesting and motivating; it can promote attention, active participation, and verbal and nonverbal responses. A number of researchers have examined the effect of musical activities on cognition, communication, and the social and sensory development of children with autism. Music appears to have a strong effect in the treatment of autism regardless of its purpose or how it is used for a particular symptom.

As a music therapist for children with autism and an autism-specialized researcher, I highly recommend using music and musical experiences in the children's daily life and treatment.

Well-designed and facilitated musical experiences can add greater things in our lives. This book discusses the influence of music on speech and language development in children with autism. It reviews recent research literature on the perception and production of speech and music in children with autism, and explains the common principles and mechanisms of music and speech perception and production in the children. The results of my original study might provide evidence for the use of music as an effective way to enhance speech production in children with ASD. In addition, I hope my clinical experiences and suggested protocols in developmental speech and language training for children with ASD in this book will augment resources for music therapy practice in treating autism and other related conditions.

Introduction

Purpose of this book

This book discusses the influence of music on speech and language development in children with ASD in terms of its research and practice. It reviews and synthesizes research literature on the perception and production of speech and music in children with autism. It provides critical resources for generating the scientific principles and mechanisms of music and speech perception and production in children with autism. The unique feature of this book is the establishment of both theoretical and clinical implications of the effects of music on speech production in children with ASD. This book provides evidence for the use of music as an effective way of enhancing speech production, and validates the clinical application utilizing musical elements to train speech production for children with ASD. With specific clinical implications and music therapy intervention protocols, this book can be used as a textbook and/or clinical manual for professionals who work with children with autism. Parents of children with ASD may find the clinical implications presented pertinent to their children's needs, enhancing their children's social communicative behaviors, particularly the conventional use of speech with their parents or caregivers. Parents might use the developmental speech and language training tool in this book in order to teach more vocabulary words and social communication skills at home.

Theoretical contribution

Music can be an effective tool for the development of language and speech skills as well as nonverbal communication skills. Music is closely related in human beings to speech and language, both neurologically and developmentally. The discussion and explanation in this book may augment the understanding of the perception and production of both music and speech. The link between music and speech is verified, and the common principles and the mechanisms of both music and speech production are explained. Furthermore, the book addresses the significance of integrating the two domains, music and speech, in early childhood development. As part of the same developmental sequence, music and speech are complementary and may reciprocate in many ways.

Researchers have theorized that musical skill and speech develop in parallel fashion from adjacent areas of the brain. This parallel in neuro-anatomy underlies the fact that both music and speech are aural forms of communication. Music and speech share the same acoustic and auditory parameters, including frequency, intensity, wave forms and timbre, duration, rate, contour, rhythm, and cadential factors. This book supports these theories by exploring basic similarities between music and speech production mechanisms. Researchers have agreed that music is perceived and produced in patterns, such as pitch, melodic contour, rhythm, and form (see Chapter 3). Music perception and production follow the principles of Gestalt perceptual organization. Pattern perception and production are also a common phenomenon for speech and language. Therefore, this book includes a discussion of the studies examining whether perception and production of elements of music is similar to perception and production of linguistic information in speech.

Music and speech serve different functions in aural communication and expression as embedded in the neuro-anatomical structures of the human brain. They might arise in parallel, but differentiate into what are called speech language and music language. Speech is more functional and concrete; music is more aesthetic and abstract. This book concludes that perception and production of musical elements through listening and singing influence speech production by activating the common mechanisms involved in both music and speech. Functional and concrete speech (vocabulary words) will be integrated into singing, and the musical elements in songs may facilitate speech production. The theoretical implication in this book could support a developmental speech and language training tool through music and expand the functions of musical elements in enhancing speech.

Clinical contribution

Investigation exploring the use of music in treating ASD has to be based on scientific evidence regarding how children with ASD perceive music. The most promising explanation for musical behaviors in autism may lie in the knowledge of brain function and perceptual processes of children with ASD. Unfortunately, resources exploring the reasons for the musical responsiveness of children with autism are limited. Therefore, empirical mechanisms of music perception and production in children with ASD as well as the theoretical foundations for the use of music in treating autism will be discussed.

With the many similarities between music and speech, educators, therapists, or parents often assume that music, and especially singing, is a valuable tool for the treatment of speech disorders. The clinical examples in this book may provide evidence of the close link between music and language development in children with ASD, and explain the similar mechanisms in their perception and production of music and speech. Once this rationale is established, the practical use of music to enhance speech and language skills in children with ASD will be discussed. The principle of music perception and production, and the scientific evidence of music's effectiveness, may justify the use of music in treating speech and language impairments in children with ASD.

The clinical implications might be useful for music therapists to implement interventions for enhancing social communicative functions for children with ASD. The clinical examples and suggested protocols will enhance the collaborative efforts of speech and language pathologists, special education teachers, and music therapists who practice speech and language training for children with ASD. A selection of materials and interventions based on scientific evidence will allow the therapists or teachers to produce more consistent and positive outcomes by the systematic implementation.

Furthermore, this book provides an example of utilizing musical elements in teaching functional vocabulary words for children with ASD. Singing has been used to teach pre-academic concepts such as the alphabet, numbers, or colors for typically developing children. The examples of music therapy intervention and/or protocols expand the functions of singing for teaching new vocabulary words and improving overall aspects of speech production in children with ASD including their semantics, pragmatics, phonology, and prosody. The clinical implication of the use of musical elements is then related to improvement in speech production of children with ASD.

A music therapy technique called developmental speech and language training through music (DSLM) is introduced as a primary method to enhance communication skills in children with ASD. "Developmental speech and language training through music is designed to utilize musical as well as related materials to enhance and facilitate speech and language development in children with developmental speech and language delays" (Thaut 2005, p.173). Therapeutic musical experiences in DSLM may range from simple singing exercises to connecting sounds or pictures with words to elicit the proper vocal production of the target words. Structurally and functionally organized music experiences of DSLM may enhance speech production, vocabulary acquisition, and social communication skills in children with ASD.

Throughout the music therapy interventions such as DSLM, children with ASD can learn functional vocabulary words that they can use effectively in everyday interactions. In addition, the children might improve various speech elements such as semantics, pragmatics, phonology, and prosody. These learning experiences and positive changes in their speech production might result in improved communication skills, more conversations, and enhanced interactions with others. Improved relationships with others and increased social-communicative experiences might help the children to gain more cognitive stimulation for optimal development and independence. Furthermore, improved semantic or phonology skills may help children to acquire reading skills.

The goals of this book are, first, validation of the clinical application utilizing musical elements to train adequate speech production for children with ASD by providing a theoretical foundation and scientific evidence for the use of music in speech and language training for the children; second, clinical application of a carefully designed program of speech and language training through music which might utilize unimpaired ability to perceive music stimuli in children with ASD and facilitate their processes of speech production; and third, education on the effect of music on speech production in children with ASD explained by the inherent structure of music stimuli and the intact capacity of pattern perception and production in children with ASD.

Autism spectrum disorders

ASD is a complex developmental disability that typically appears during the first three years of life and currently affects 1 in every 110 American children. ASD is identified as a behaviorally defined syndrome with a broad range of severity, resulting from brain dysfunction. The diagnostic schemes and description of the underlying deficits in ASD have evolved and changed since Leo Kanner's first description of infantile autism in 1943. One criterion for diagnosis has remained constant: difficulty in the development of social communication. In particular, speech and language impairment has been regarded as one of the most significant deficits in persons with ASD. Effective intervention therefore is needed in the development of social communication including speech and language.

Social communication requires the acquisition and use of conventional and socially appropriate means to communicate for a variety of purposes across social contexts (Prizant and Wetherby 2005). Communication may include verbal and nonverbal behaviors, such as language expressed through speech, identifying pictures, gestures, or manual signs. In particular, communicative language competence may determine the extent to which individuals with ASD can develop relationships with others and participate in daily activities at school, at home, and in the community. Furthermore, social communication ability, specifically the use of language, is critical for individuals with ASD to lead independent and productive lives.

The level of communicative language competence achieved by children with ASD is closely related to their development of cognitive, emotional, and social behaviors. In addition, gains in communication skills are directly related to the prevention and reduction of problem behaviors in children with ASD. Furthermore, a delay in the development of speech and language is one of the most distinguishable deficits in children with ASD, compared to typically developing children. Parents of children with autism have identified speech and language impairment as one of the most significant stresses they experience with their children in the preschool and school years. In summary, a deficit in the communicative use of language is a defining feature of ASD, and it directly reflects the core developmental difficulties of children with ASD. Social communication ability is the key for success in everyday activities for children with ASD. Providing an effective intervention to improve communication skills and language is a high priority in efforts to treat children with ASD.

Need for effective interventions and treatments for communication deficits in ASD

Communication difficulties typically are compounded by significant impairments in social interaction and appropriate behaviors. Researchers state that children may use aberrant behaviors for communication purposes when they lack the appropriate skills to communicate (Chung *et al.* 1995;

Sigafoos 2000). To address both the communication and behavioral needs of children with ASD, researchers and practitioners have investigated numerous interventions and treatment approaches. Intervention or treatment approaches for enhancing social communication abilities for children with ASD vary greatly, and they range in a continuum from traditional discrete trials, to more contemporary behavioral approaches that utilize naturalistic language teaching techniques, to developmental approaches (Goldstein 2002; Paul and Sutherland 2005; Prizant and Wetherby 1993; Wetherby and Woods 2008).

The National Research Council (NRC 2001) recommended that educational approaches should address the core deficits faced by children with ASD, and that meaningful outcome measures must address two areas: first, gains in initiation of spontaneous communication in functional activities; and second, generalization of gains across activities, interactions (adult and peer), and environments. The NRC also identified six instructional priorities which include: (1) functional, spontaneous communication; (2) social instruction in various settings; (3) teaching of play skills focusing on appropriate use of toys and play with peers; (4) instruction leading to generalization and maintenance of cognitive goals in natural contexts; (5) positive approaches to address problem behaviors; and (6) functional academic skills when appropriate (NRC 2001; Prizant and Wetherby 2005). Collectively, social communication and functional language abilities are regarded as the most critical areas to address in supporting the development of individuals with ASD, and it is also critical to develop and implement effective interventions which fulfill the instructional priorities.

Use of music in speech and language training for children with ASD

Music has been commonly used in autism treatment as a behavioral and developmental method because music is interesting and motivating. It can promote attention, active participation, and verbal and nonverbal responses. A number of researchers have examined the effect of musical activities on cognition, communication, and the social and sensory development of children with autism (Brownell 2002; Buday 1995; Hoskins 1988; Kaplan and Steele 2005; Lim 2010; Thaut 1999; Whipple 2004). Music therapy appears to be an effective approach to address a variety of purposes and symptoms in the treatment of autism including language and communication skills, social skills, cognitive skills, and behavioral skills. Whipple (2004) indicated that all types of music intervention, including singing, background music, social stories set to music, and following directions in music, have been effective for children and adolescents with autism. In almost every treatment approach for communication deficits in children with autism or other developmental disabilities, music has been used as a consistent and reliable way to facilitate speech and language and develop communication skills.

When I examined the effect of DSLM on the speech production of fifty children with ASD, I found that children with ASD appear to perceive important linguistic information embedded in music stimuli which are organized by principles of pattern perception, and that children are in turn able to produce the words as functional speech (Lim 2010). These results provide evidence for the use of music as an effective way to enhance speech production in children with ASD. The effect of music on speech production in children with ASD might be explained by the inherent structure of music stimuli and the intact capacity of pattern perception and production in children with ASD. Results suggest that carefully designed age-appropriate music interventions can provide a rich opportunity for productive communication experiences in children with ASD.

Researchers suggest that music could be an effective part of intervention for children with ASD for three reasons: first, some children with ASD have musical sensitivity; second, children with ASD may have a perceptual preference for music; and third, some children with ASD are able to produce musical patterns.

Musical sensitivity in children with ASD

Musical sensitivity refers to a particular capacity of responsiveness to musical stimuli. A distinctive sensitivity and attention to music has been frequently mentioned in the literature on children with ASD. Musical sensitivity in children with ASD includes auditory acuity such as superior auditory detection or discrimination abilities and strong memory for melodies. Early studies on music and children with autism focused on the unique ways that children with ASD respond to music. In the early 1950s, Sherwin reported three case studies with boys with autism who showed unusual auditory sensitivity, perfect pitch, strong melodic memory, and great interest in playing musical instruments (Sherwin 1953). Other autism researchers have reported the exceptional ability in piano performance of children with autism (Applebaum *et al.* 1979; O'Connell 1974). These reports indicate that some children with autism have an unusual and superior musical sensitivity.

Not all children with autism, however, possess such musical sensitivity or a particular musical ability. Furthermore, it is not known that musical ability transfers to functional behaviors for children with autism. In fact, cognitive or functional ability does not relate to their superior auditory acuity and musical sensitivity (Berger 2002; O'Connell 1974; Radocy and Boyle 2003). Some children with ASD who have perfect pitch showed limited expressive language (Berger 2002; O'Connell 1974). In addition, they showed surprising and inappropriate behaviors, such as screaming when a piece of music happened to be played in a different key, not the original key which was first presented (Berger 2002).

Perceptual preference for music in children with ASD

Another reason why music may play an effective role in the speech and language development of children with ASD is their perceptual preference of music. Children with autism are more likely to attend to an auditory than to a visual stimulus, especially when the auditory stimulus is musical (Kolko, Anderson and Campbell 1980; Thaut 1987). Thaut (1987) found that when given a choice children with ASD showed a slight preference for the musical stimulus when comparing this response to visual stimuli. Children with autism spent a significantly longer amount of time listening to the music than watching the visual stimulus. A group of non-autistic children matched by approximate chronological age and developmental age, however, preferred the visual stimulus over the music. An earlier study on music and children with autism compared the auditory preferences of children with and without autism. In the study, typical children showed no preference, whereas children with autism preferred music when given a listening choice between verbal and musical selections (Blackstock 1978). These findings might indicate that there is a marked difference in preference and response to music between children with and without autism.

Production of musical patterns by children with ASD

Some studies have indicated that, although children with ASD have sensory and cognitive deficits, they are able to perceive and produce musical patterns (Edgerton 1994; Thaut 1988; Lim 2010). Many children with autism perform well musically in comparison with other areas of their behaviors, as well as in comparison with children without autism. Frith

(1972) compared sequences of either musical tones or colors spontaneously produced by children with autism, those with intellectual disabilities, or typical children. Musical tone sequences produced by children with autism were more complex and varied to a significant degree, and thus superior to the musical tones of children without autism as well as to their color sequences (Frith 1972).

Improvised musical tone sequences produced by children with autism were compared with musical improvisations by typical children and children with intellectual disabilities (Thaut 1988). Improvised melodies produced by children with autism were similar to those of normally developing children. Children with autism scored significantly higher than children with intellectual disabilities on rhythm production, restriction (i.e. maintaining musical rules), originality, and total performance score. Thaut (1988) reported that, on the given musical performance test, children with autism did not perform significantly lower than normally developing children.

In summary, the reviewed studies demonstrate that many children with ASD have superior musical sensitivity and a perceptual preference for music. Research has shown that sometimes these children respond more favorably and appropriately to music than other sensory stimuli. Furthermore, children with ASD are able to perceive and produce well-organized musical patterns, such as melodic and rhythmic patterns. Development of speech and language also depends largely on pattern perception and production. Therefore, children with ASD who have intact musical abilities might influence the perception and production of patterns in speech and language. It is worthwhile to examine the effects of music on speech and language development in children with ASD, and the next section discusses the effect of music therapy on the non-musical skills of children with ASD, in particular the therapeutic effect of music on communicative behaviors including speech and language.

General effects of music therapy on autism spectrum disorders

Since 1965, a number of researchers have examined the effect of musical activities on the cognitive, social, and sensory development of children with ASD. A meta-analysis and a descriptive analysis have both explored the general effects of music therapy interventions on individuals with ASD (Kaplan and Steele 2003; Whipple 2004). One researcher analyzed nine quantitative studies comparing music to non-music conditions during the treatment of children and adolescents with autism (Whipple 2004). Results indicated that all types of music intervention, including singing, background music, social stories set to music, and following directions in music, have been effective for children and adolescents with autism. According to the analysis, benefits from the use of music therapy included increased appropriate social behaviors such as engagement with others, and decreased stereotypical and self-stimulatory behaviors. In particular, the use of music interventions was effective in increased communicative behaviors including vocalization, verbalization, gestures, vocabulary comprehension, and echolalia with communicative intention.

Kaplan and Steele (2003) conducted a descriptive study with forty autistic patients treated over a two-year period. They found that the primary goal areas in music therapy intervention for children with ASD were language and communication. In addition, the most frequently utilized interventions were interactive singing and interactive instrument playing. The most common type of session for music therapy interventions was individual, which utilized the direct interaction between therapist and client. The analysis also revealed that a variety of music therapy interventions were effective across a number of different treatment goals, such as behavioral and psychosocial, language and communication, perceptual and motor, and cognitive and musical goals. In other words, all types of interventions were equally effective for general enhancement of functioning in individuals with ASD. Moreover, parents and caregivers of children with ASD reported that their children applied and generalized skills or responses acquired in music therapy to non-music therapy environments. The researchers, however, did not provide an explanation of how those skills or responses transferred to non-musical functions in children with ASD.

While these analyses indicated that music therapy is effective across a number of functioning domains for individuals with ASD, several critical limitations can be noted in these bodies of research. The benefits of music were not differentiated by treatment intervention, age of participants, selection of music, or goal areas (Kaplan and Steele 2005; Whipple 2004). These studies emphasized the general effects of music on autism and also mentioned a strong beneficial effect of music on speech and language development of children with ASD; however, the studies did not indicate a theoretical paradigm and did not explain how music impacts behaviors in individuals with ASD. More clinical studies providing the rational connection between music therapy interventions and the positive outcomes are necessary.

The positive effects of music on speech and language development in ASD

Some of the early music therapy literature focused specifically on the effect of music on communication and language improvement in children with speech and language delays, including children with ASD. Stevens and Clark (1969) examined the effect of music therapy on socially adaptive behaviors and communication among children with autism. Results indicated that music therapy techniques such as instrument playing, singing, or action songs were found to be significantly effective in improving social and communicative behaviors of children with autism including interpersonal verbal or nonverbal communication; involvement; and drive for mastery (Stevens and Clark 1969).

Other researchers found that the use of contingent music and corresponding audiovisual stimuli significantly increased the frequency of verbal production including general intelligible and spontaneous speech in children with speech and language delay (Seybold 1971; Walker 1972). Listening to music and playing rhythm instruments appeared to have reward value for the participants. When pleasurable and varied stimuli are paired with appropriate verbal behavior, learning may be enhanced for children with speech and language impairments. Seybold (1971) suggested that music activities in speech therapy provided the necessary stimulation for speech-delayed children to use spontaneous speech. Researchers also speculated that the positive effect of music on increased spontaneous speech might be the result of the pleasurable experience associated with music and a more comfortable atmosphere created by the musical experience.

In more recent music and autism literature, similar results have been reported regarding the positive effect of music on speech and language in children with ASD. Antiphonal singing with picture cards resulted in a significant improvement in expressive and receptive language in children with autism (Hoskins 1988).[1] A combination of manual signs and singing elicited a significantly higher number of signs and spoken words imitated by children with autism, in comparison to signs and spoken words imitated during a speech-only condition (Buday 1995). Brownell (2002) reported that the use of a musically adapted social story was an effective and viable

---

1   Antiphonal singing refers to singing in response. In Hoskins's (1988) study, a music therapist led the group in antiphonal singing: a picture of an object was shown to the group, and the therapist sang a three-to-five-word phrase about the object. The group then repeated the object name with the therapist.

treatment option for modifying behaviors in children with autism, such as excessive delayed echolalia, following directions, or using a quiet voice in the classroom. These findings suggest a link between music and speech and language development in children with ASD.

The reviewed studies investigated more specific outcomes of music's effect on communication and speech and language development in children with ASD. The positive effects for music in these studies were largely attributed to increased attention, enjoyment, and optimal social context (Brownell 2002; Buday 1995; Seybold 1971; Walker 1972). The previous studies, however, did not describe the scientific mechanisms by which music can impact the speech and language of children with ASD. Furthermore, methods and outcomes were not clearly stated in certain studies. Research is needed to explore the effect of a systematic intervention on speech and language skills in children with ASD. Such an intervention should be based on scientific evidence regarding the unique ways in which children with ASD perceive and produce music. Research regarding the influence of music on speech and language development in ASD should describe the mechanisms of music perception and production in this population. In addition, such research should explore similarities between perception and production of music and speech and language in ASD. This kind of research will explore how music can mediate change in the communicative behaviors in children with ASD.

Most recently, I examined the effect of music as part of developmental speech and language training for children with ASD (Lim 2010). This study compared the effect of training conditions—music, speech, and no-training—on the verbal production of children with ASD. Participants were fifty children with ASD, age range three to five years, who had previously been evaluated on standard tests of language and level of functioning. Eighteen participants in music training watched a music video containing six songs and pictures of the thirty-six target words or two-word phrases, and eighteen participants in speech training watched a speech video containing six stories and pictures of the target words/phrases. Fourteen participants were randomly assigned to a no-training condition. Both high and low functioning participants improved their speech production after receiving either music or speech training; however, low functioning participants showed a greater improvement after the music training than the speech training. The study indicates that children with ASD perceive important linguistic information embedded in music stimuli organized by principles of pattern perception, and produce the functional speech (Lim

2010). My study, however, did not use standardized language tests to examine the effect of music on speech production. In order to generalize the effect on the speech and language development in children with ASD, such investigations using a standardized speech and language evaluation tool with a careful external validity control might be needed.

In conclusion, speech and language impairments have been regarded as one of the most pervasive developmental deficits in children with ASD. A number of studies have suggested that music can positively influence treatment of these deficits, due to musical sensitivity, preference, and perceptual abilities in children with autism.

PART I

Use of Music in Speech and Language Training for Children with ASD

Research and Scientific Evidence

1

Speech and Language Impairments in Children with ASD

Inadequate use of language is a defining feature of ASD. Most parents of autistic children first begin to be concerned that something is not quite right in their child's development when early delay or regression occurs in the development of speech. Many studies which focused on the language of verbal children with ASD identified aberrant speech features, such as unusual word choice, pronoun reversal, echolalia, incoherent discourse, unresponsiveness to questions, aberrant prosody, and lack of drive to communicate (Rapin and Dunn 2003). Persistent lack of speech of some individuals with ASD was attributed to the severity of their disorders, and attendant intellectual disabilities, rather than possible inability to decode auditory language. These studies determined that production and comprehension of speech was more severely compromised in children with ASD than children with intellectual disabilities matched for nonverbal cognitive level (Lord and Paul 1997).

Characteristics of speech and language in children with autism

By age three, most children have passed predictable milestones on the path to learning language; one of the earliest is babbling. By their first birthday, typical toddlers say a word or two, turn and look when they hear their name, point when they want a toy, and, when offered something undesirable, make it clear that the answer is "No." These communication skills are usually severely impaired in children with autism. What the individual understands (receptive language) as well as what is actually spoken by the individual (expressive language) are significantly delayed or nonexistent. Deficits in language comprehension include the inability to understand simple directions, questions, or commands. There may be an absence of dramatic or pretend play and these children may not be able to engage in simple age-appropriate childhood games such as Simon Says or Hide-and-Go-Seek. Teens and adults with autism may continue to engage in playing games that are age inappropriate. Children with autism who do speak may be unable to initiate or participate in a two-way conversation (reciprocal). Their speech may seem to lack the normal emotion and sound flat or monotonous. The sentences are often very immature: "Want water" instead of "I want some water please." Children with autism often repeat words or phrases that are spoken to them. For example, you might say "Look at the train!" and the child or adult may respond "train," without any knowledge of what was said. This repetition is known as echolalia. Memorization and recitation of songs, stories, commercials, or even entire scripts is not uncommon. While many feel this is a sign of intelligence, some children with autism do not appear to understand any of the content in their speech.

About a third to a half of individuals with autism do not develop enough natural speech to meet their daily communication needs. Differences in communication may be present from the first year of life, and may include delayed onset of babbling, unusual gestures, diminished responsiveness, and vocal patterns that are not synchronized with the caregiver. In the second and third years, children with autism have less frequent and less diverse babbling, consonants, words, and word combinations; their gestures are often less integrated with words. Some people with autism remain mute throughout their lives; although the majority develops spoken language and all eventually learn to communicate in some way. Some infants who show signs of autism "coo" and babble during the first few months of life, but later stop. Others may be delayed, developing language as late as ages five to nine. Some children may learn to use communication systems such as picture communication, basic sign language, or voice output devices.

Children with autism who do speak often use language in unusual ways. They seem unable to combine words into meaningful sentences. Some speak only single words, while others repeat the same phrase over and over. They may repeat or copy what they hear, as in echolalia. Although many children with autism go through a stage where they repeat what they hear, it normally passes by the time they are three. Children with autism are less likely to make requests or share experiences, and are more likely to simply repeat others' words or reverse pronouns. Children with autism may have difficulty with imaginative play and with developing symbols into language.

Some children with autism who are only mildly affected may exhibit slight delays in language, or even seem to have precocious language and unusually large vocabularies, but have great difficulty in sustaining a conversation. The "give and take" of normal conversations may be hard, although they may often obsessively carry on a monologue on a favorite subject, giving others little opportunity to comment. Another common difficulty is the inability to understand body language, tone of voice, or prosody of speech. For example, someone with autism might interpret a sarcastic expression such as "Oh, that's just great" as meaning it really is great.

While it can be challenging for others to understand what children with autism are saying, their body language may also be difficult to understand. Facial expressions, movements, and gestures may not match what they are saying. Their tone of voice may fail to reflect their feelings. They may use a high pitched, or flat, electronically or artificially generated voice. Some children demonstrate relatively good concrete language skills like adults' speech; however, they tend to fail to pick up on the "kid-speak" that is common in their peers. Without meaningful gestures or the language to ask for things, children with autism are less able to let others know what they need. As a result, the children may use aberrant behaviors for communication purposes when they lack the appropriate skills to communicate. As they grow up, they can become increasingly aware of their difficulties in understanding others and in being understood. They are at greater risk of becoming anxious or depressed. Communication difficulties typically are compounded by significant impairments in social interaction and appropriate behaviors.

Clinical research findings for speech and language impairments in children with ASD

Various studies support the view that the language disorders of children with ASD have much in common with those of children with developmental language disorders or specific language impairment (SLI) (Tager-Flusberg 2003). More specifically, there was a subgroup of children with autism who also had SLI. Language impairment is a co-occurring disorder in some, but not all, children with autism. This subgroup of children with autism shared the same phenotypic features of language impairment or abnormal speech that characterize SLI, such as similar patterns of atypical brain asymmetry. The language disorders with autism, however, differ strikingly by their universally impaired pragmatics, including problems with the conversational use of language, and the comprehension of discourse (Rapin and Dunn 2003; Tager-Flusberg 2003).

Tager-Flusberg (1981, 2003) indicated that children with ASD do not differ from children with intellectual disabilities in phonology or syntax, but they have more severe comprehension and pragmatic deficits than children with developmental language disorders. Rapin and Dunn (2003) indicated that children with ASD also differ by the prevalence of higher order processing disorders such as lexical or syntactic impairments, and of impaired semantic classification of words. Rapin and Dunn (2003) suggested that these deficits may be ascribed to problems with semantic organization, rather than to delayed maturation of phonology and syntax. Children with ASD also have word retrieval deficit, which is semantic in nature due to impaired comprehension and formulating of discourse (Rapin and Dunn 2003). In addition, many children with ASD are quite devoid of speech affect or prosody (Tager-Flusberg 1997). In summary, children with ASD frequently have various kinds of language deficits; however, semantic, pragmatic, and prosody deficits are the most pervasive.

In spite of these deficits, more than half of all children with ASD show an intact ability to perceive and produce speech sounds, and do develop some level of functional speech (Schuler 1995; Tager-Flusberg 1997). Children with ASD clearly have language impairments; however, they also have certain components of language that are intact (Paul and Sutherland 2005; Prizant and Wetherby 2005; Tager-Flusberg 1997). Studies have shown that children with autism who do develop some functional language have relatively little difficulty acquiring the formal, rule-governed components of language, such as phonology and syntax. By contrast, certain pragmatic aspects of language, those that entail an understanding of others' minds, are specifically and uniquely impaired in autism (Tager-Flusberg 1997).

Tager-Flusberg (1997) identified examples of impaired and not impaired (spared) components of language and communication in autism. Speech sounds (i.e. phonology), linguistic form (i.e. syntax), questions for requests, turn-taking abilities, and communicative gestures are usually spared in children with ASD. However, intonation and vocal quality (i.e. prosody), linguistic function (i.e. pragmatics), semantics, questions seeking information, adding to a conversational topic, and expressive gestures are usually impaired.

Early clinical descriptions of autistic language focused on its atypical characteristics: echolalia, pronoun reversals, use of stereotyped language, and unusual meanings (Kanner 1946). Some early researchers went on to argue that even the process of communication development was different in autism; that is, children with autism who acquire language do not follow the same stages or developmental patterns as do other children (as cited in Tager-Flusberg 1997). More recent studies, however, have demonstrated that children with ASD exhibit much greater similarity to other children without autism. They acquire more of the computational and semantic aspects of language than was previously thought.

Tager-Flusberg *et al.* (1990) conducted a longitudinal study with six children with ASD and found that they followed the same developmental path as children with Down syndrome who were being compared as part of the study, and as typically developing children drawn from the extant literature. In looking at their grammatical development, children with autism and those with Down syndrome showed similar growth curves in the length of their utterances. For most of the children with autism, however, the rate of growth was slower than in normally developing children. The researchers also found that children with ASD and Down syndrome acquired grammatical structures in the same order as normally developing children (Tager-Flusberg and Calkins 1990; Tager-Flusberg *et al.* 1990).

More detailed analysis of the development patterns and a comparison of spontaneous and imitative (or echolalic) utterances suggested that even the processes involved in grammatical development in the children with ASD were similar to those of typically developing children (Tager-Flusberg and Calkins 1990). Other longitudinal studies indicated that the lexical growth (i.e. vocabulary learning) and semantic representations of children with ASD also showed a developmental pattern similar to typically developing children (Tager-Flusberg 1985, 1986). The development of word use is also similar to children without autism, but it is slower (Travis and Sigman 2001). Children with autism who acquire speech follow the same pattern that typically developing children do, but at a reduced rate (Paul and Sutherland 2005).

Children with ASD assign words to the same conceptual categories as typically developing children do (Lord and Paul 1997; Paul and Sutherland 2005). For example, children with ASD recognize objects they sit on as "chairs." High functioning children with autism use semantic groupings (e.g. bird, boat, food) in ways that are very similar to those used by non-autistic children to categorize and to retrieve words (Boucher 1988; Lord and Paul 1997; Minshew and Goldstein 1993; Tager-Flusberg 1985). In fact, some high functioning individuals with ASD show particular interest in words. Unusual and idiosyncratic word use, such as inventing words, is frequently seen (Volden and Lord 1991). Tager-Flusberg (1991) suggests that children with autism are able to represent word meanings in memory, but fail to use these meanings in a conventional way in retrieval or organizational tasks.

Abnormal auditory cortical processing in children with ASD

Some researchers suggest that delayed speech development in children with ASD is due to problems or deficits in the neural mechanisms for the perception and production of sounds (Rapin and Dunn 2003). Autism may be associated with abnormal auditory behavior, and abnormal perception of speech-like sounds in childhood may account for inadequate responses to sounds, and thus for language impairments typical of ASD (Boddaert et al. 2004).

Roberts et al. (2008) reported that the brains of children with ASD react to sounds a fraction of a second slower than those of normal children. In their study, thirty children with ASD aged 6–15 listened to a battery of sound and syllables while monitoring the tiny magnetic fields produced by the brain's electrical impulses using a technique called magnetoencephalography (MEG). Since a single syllable in a multisyllable word might take less than one-quarter of a second to say, the researchers found that one-twentieth of a second extra delay in the response time of the brains of children with autism may hamper their ability to comprehend speech language. The study concluded that there could be abnormal routing or a lack of connectivity in the brains of children with ASD. Microscopic examination of the brain tissue of individuals with autism has shown there may be fewer connections between their brain cells (Roberts et al. 2008). The results of the study might provide strong supporting evidence for the emerging theory that speech and language deficit in autism is a problem of connectivity in the brain.

Rapin and Dunn (2003) found that children with autism who show communication or language deficits had decreased glucose metabolism in the lateral temporal gyri bilaterally compared to typically developing children. The lateral temporal gyri are cortical areas crucial to auditory and language processing. Some cortical evoked response studies provide evidence for more consistent dysfunction in the lateral surface of the superior temporal gyrus. A persistent abnormality in the secondary auditory cortex (i.e. auditory associative area) has been found in children with ASD (Rapin and Dunn 2003).

Boddaert *et al.* (2003) studied auditory cortical processing in adults with autism using complex speech-like sounds. They found less activation of the left hemisphere temporal word processing network in adults with autism than in healthy comparison participants. The results obtained for autistic adults suggest a dysfunction of specific temporal regions specializing in the perception and integration of complex sounds. Consequently, such auditory stimuli are rarely recognized as speech. The abnormal pattern of activation found in adults with autism could reflect basic anomalies of paralinguistic auditory processing, rather than a consequence of abnormal language development.

More recently, Boddaert *et al.* (2004) conducted a positron emission tomography (PET) auditory activation study to investigate whether the abnormal cortical-auditory processing is also present in children with ASD. They found significant activation of the auditory cortex in the bilateral superior temporal gyrus in both children with ASD and children with intellectual disabilities while children were listening to speech-like stimuli. However, the activation pattern was different for the two groups. The children with intellectual disabilities showed activation of the superior temporal cortex bilaterally with left-biased asymmetry, as the investigators have previously observed in normal adults. This left dominance, however, was not observed in the children with ASD. In addition, children with autism had additional significant activation outside the auditory cortex, including the left temporal pole, the bilateral cingulum, the bilateral posterior parietal, the cerebellar hemispheres, and the brain stem. The direct comparison between the two groups of children revealed less activation in left speech-related areas, including Wernicke's area, in autistic children. The abnormal cortical activities in children with ASD are similar to those previously described in adults with autism (Boddaert *et al.* 2004).

The researchers concluded that listening to complex speech sounds induced an abnormal cortical activation including an aberrant functioning network in children with ASD (Boddaert *et al.* 2004). This abnormal auditory-cortical activation might be associated with a dysfunction of specific temporal regions specialized in the perception and the integration of complex sounds. The areas found to be less activated by complex sounds in children with ASD are thought to be auditory association areas that are involved in word processing and are also presumed to act as an interface between word perception and long-term representation of familiar words in memory (Price *et al.* 1996; Wise *et al.* 2001). In the dominant hemisphere for language, these areas play a critical role in the ability to understand and produce meaningful speech. Thus, a dysfunction of left speech-related cortical areas could be the origin of the language developmental impairments observed in autism.

Many previous studies suggest that speech and language impairments in autism are behavior problems or learning disabilities. The reviewed literature regarding abnormal auditory cortical processing in children with ASD indicates that the origin of speech and language deficits may be brain dysfunction. Despite this brain dysfunction, a number of studies about speech and language development in ASD indicate that children with ASD can still learn language and develop their communication skills through speech. Researchers suggest focusing on the children's spared capacity for language development and exploring ways to facilitate their functional speech (Lord and Paul 1997; Prizant and Wetherby 2005).

2

Perception and Production of Speech in Children with ASD

Language acquisition in children with ASD: development of functional speech

Echolalia

One of the most salient examples of deviant speech in autism is echolalia, the repetition of utterance with a similar intonation of words or phrases that someone else has said. Echolalia may occur immediately after or significantly later than the original production of an utterance (Lord and Paul 1997; Prizant and Wetherby 2005; Rydell and Prizant 1995). Immediate echolalia is produced either following immediately, or within two turns of the original production, and involves exact repetition (i.e. pure echolalia) or minimal structural changes (i.e. mitigated immediate echolalia). Immediate echolalia has been considered a necessary stage of language development for verbal children with autism (Prizant and Duchan 1981). Delayed echolalia is repeated at a significantly later time (i.e. at least three turns following the original utterance, but more typically hours, days, or even weeks later), and also involves exact repetition, or minimal structural changes. The production process of delayed echolalia involves retrieval of information from some type of long-term memory, while for immediate echolalia, short-term memory is most often implicated.

Echolalia is characteristic of at least 85 percent of the children with ASD who acquire speech (Prizant 1987; Rydell and Prizant 1995), and was once viewed as an undesirable, nonfunctional communication behavior (Koegel, Lovaas and Schreibman 1974; Lovaas 1977). Some researchers considered echolalia a type of communication disorder and therefore advocated for the extinction or replacement of echolalic behaviors through the use of behavior modification procedures (Lovaas 1977). Some researchers defined echolalia as a pathological behavior that could interfere with cognitive and linguistic growth (Coleman and Stedman 1974; Schreibman and Carr 1978). Other clinical researchers, however, beginning with Fay (1969) and elaborated by Prizant and colleagues (Prizant 1983; Prizant and Duchan 1981), have emphasized that immediate and delayed echolalia have functions for children with ASD (Lim 2010; Lord and Paul 1997; Paul and Sutherland 2005; Prizant and Wetherby 1993, 2005; Sundberg and Partington 1998). These researchers describe echolalia as serving communicative functions, and explain echolalic behavior within the context of a child's cognitive and linguistic development.

Prizant and Duchan (1981) conducted a study to discover how immediate echolalia functioned for children with ASD in interacting with familiar adults. After conducting a multilevel analysis of over a thousand utterances from four children with autism who produced echolalic speech, Prizant and Duchan (1981) concluded that immediate echolalia is not a meaningless behavior or undesirable symptom. The results indicated that for all four children in the study, regardless of individual communicative functioning levels, the percentage of echolalia produced with evidence of comprehension (62.75%) was significantly greater than the percentage produced with no evidence of comprehension (37.25%). Prizant and Duchan (1981) identified six communicative functions of immediate echolalia: turn-taking, assertions, affirmative answers, requests, rehearsal to aid processing, and self-regulation. In summary, echolalia has been reevaluated as a developmental behavior that might accomplish communicative purposes.

Prizant (1983) further hypothesized that echolalic behavior may play a role in the acquisition of linguistic function and structure of speech among children with autism. Tager-Flusberg (1985, p.72) stated, "Echolalia and stereotyped language are now seen as primitive strategies for communicating, especially in the context of poor comprehension." Echolalia is regarded as a speech imitation skill, and this particular speech production may predict further speech-communication development in children with ASD.

Goldstein (2002) conducted a meta-analysis of studies in communication interventions for children with ASD. The participants who benefit most from the interventions (e.g. modeling, prompting, fading, or use of visual modality) seem to have better verbal imitation skills. Furthermore, children with good verbal imitation skills (i.e. echolalia) are more likely to demonstrate speech production in addition to or in lieu of sign production than children with poor verbal skills. These findings suggest that a positive correlation might exist between imitation skills of children with ASD and their communication development. Children with ASD may learn communication behavior including functional use of speech through imitation.

Imitating and copying patterns in a partner's gestures, sequential movements, and behaviors are key predictors of language outcome in children with ASD. Imitation may be a developmental precursor of communicative behaviors for children with autism (Charman and Baron-Cohen 1994; Charman *et al.* 2003; Paul and Sutherland 2005). Charman and Baron-Cohen (1994) found that children with autism have an intact ability to imitate a basic level of gestures and procedures (i.e. sequential behaviors). Their performance did not differ from that of children with intellectual disabilities, and suggests that children with ASD have some ability to imitate patterns. Charman *et al.* (2003) conducted a longitudinal study with nine children with autism and nine children with pervasive developmental disorders (PDD) to examine associations between diagnosis, joint attention, play and imitation abilities, and language outcome. Charman *et al.* (2003) demonstrated that imitation of actions on objects at age 20 months was associated with language ability at four years. Results confirmed that both joint attention and imitation were longitudinal predictors of later language ability, both receptively and expressively.

Echolalia might be one of the main predictors for the further speech and language development in ASD (Lim 2010). This finding agrees with previous studies which indicated that children with echolalia are more likely to have higher functional language development than children without echolalia (Lord and Paul 1997; Paul and Sutherland 2005; Prizant and Wetherby 1993, 2005; Sundberg and Partington 1998). Findings from previous studies suggest that echolalia serves a communicative function, and that echolalic behavior can evolve into functional speech. My own study in particular suggests that echolalic speech is related to the production of functional speech patterns and to acquisition of further functional language in children with ASD (Lim 2010). Collectively, children with ASD have an intact ability to recognize and imitate patterns in other people's gestures, sequential movements, and social-communicative behaviors. Moreover, the degree of their ability to imitate can predict the subsequent language development.

Connection between echolalia and development of functional speech

From the findings of the reviewed studies, it is possible to postulate that some children with ASD have an intact ability to recognize and imitate patterns heard in others' speech (i.e. echolalia) and other communicative behaviors (i.e. gesture and sequential movements). Prizant *et al.* (1997) suggest that 50 percent of individuals with autism and PDD develop communicative and language-related cognitive abilities; that is, they can communicate through language.

These individuals experience two general levels of language development: the emerging language level and the advanced language level (Prizant *et al.* 1997). At the first level, which is referred to as the emerging and early language level, individuals show evidence of the acquisition of a conventional symbolic system for communication. They might have expressive abilities ranging from the emergence of a stable, core vocabulary of single words used with comprehension and intent, to the production of early multiword utterances or sign-symbol combinations that demonstrate the acquisition of early semantic-syntactic knowledge. At this level, echolalia and other forms of unconventional verbal behaviors (UVB) may comprise a significant portion of expressive utterances, and may be used along with single and multiword utterances to serve different communicative functions (Prizant *et al.* 1997).

At the second level, which is referred to as the more advanced language level, individuals show abilities beyond emerging and early states of language acquisition. Their expressive language abilities range from the production of more grammatically complete simple utterances and different sentence types, to the use of language as part of a conversational and narrative discourse. They use language both expressively and receptively as a primary mode of acquiring and conveying information, and of expressing needs and desires to others. Language production at more advanced language levels may reflect a relatively sophisticated knowledge of linguistic structure (e.g. production and comprehension of different sentence types, including declaratives, questions, negatives, and even complex sentence forms), although significant difficulties in pragmatics or social use of language may still remain (Prizant *et al.* 1997; Tager-Flusberg 1997).

Collectively, emerging and advanced language levels include individuals with autism or PDD who have achieved at least a single-word utterance state in expressive linguistic ability, as well as those who are able to use language in conversations. Many autistic individuals within this range of ability also produce echolalia and other forms of unconventional verbal behavior, or have progressed through periods of echolalia in language development (Prizant and Wetherby 1993). Prizant *et al.* (1997) demonstrated that children with ASD at the emerging language level might communicate primarily through early language forms and echolalia, while children at more advanced linguistic levels might have the ability to communicate more consistently through generative and creative linguistic means. Prizant *et al.* (1997) indicated that there is a continuum of communicative ability in children with ASD at language states, rather than a clear dichotomy of language state. Progressing to advanced language levels from a single-word utterance, however, is a challenging developmental process.

At the emerging language level and even at the more advanced language level, children with ASD may produce unconventional verbal behaviors (UVB) for communicative as well as non-communicative purposes (Prizant and Wetherby 1993). Researchers pointed out that the presence of echolalia or UVB is critical for enhancing language and communication development in ASD (Prizant *et al.* 1997). Within the category of UVB, there is a continuum of linguistic behavior ranging from highly unconventional and non-interactive speech patterns to speech patterns that are produced with clear intent and are close enough to conventional forms that most listeners understand the speaker's purpose and meaning. Therefore, the communicative success of individuals at emerging language levels will vary greatly, depending on the presence of UVB and the degree of conventionality and intentionality achieved (Prizant *et al.* 1997).

Gestalt style of language development in children with ASD

Gestalt styles of language acquisition in children with ASD

Echolalia is the most common form of UVB and is the most frequently discussed characteristic of children with ASD who acquire speech (Prizant 1983). Echolalia and other UVB have been offered as evidence of Gestalt processing of language in autism (Frith 1972; Prizant 1983; Rydell and Prizant 1995). Based on a study of typical language acquisition (Peters 1983), echolalia has been referred to as a "Gestalt language form" (Prizant 1983; Prizant *et al.* 1997).

Gestalt language forms are unanalyzed units of speech. They refer to multiword utterances that are learned as memorized forms or whole units, but may appear to be the result of productive linguistic processes or the application of combinatorial rules (Prizant 1983). Gestalt language forms are directly related to a Gestalt style of language acquisition, in which early utterances are comprised largely of Gestalt forms (i.e. structures or patterns). In addition, growth and progress in the acquisition of a flexible and generative language system depends on analysis and segmentation of Gestalt forms for rule induction.[1]

In the language development of typical children, two dominant styles of acquisition have been discussed. The first style, referred to as "analytic," is one in which children in early-stage language development emphasize single words for primarily referential functions and acquire more complex language by combining elements into multiword utterances using productive rules. In the Gestalt style of language acquisition, children produce unanalyzed language forms or unanalyzed "chunks" with little appreciation of their internal structure or specific meaning, although the utterances may be used somewhat appropriately in communicative interactions (Prizant 1983). Peters (1980) claimed that typical children's use of unanalyzed chunks or deferred imitations served important functions in ongoing communicative interactions as well as in the language acquisition process.

Gestalt and analytic styles of language acquisition are not necessarily exclusive of one another. Most typical children use the analytic style, or may use both analytic and Gestalt forms (Barrett 1999; Eysenck 2001; Peters 1977, 1983; Prizant 1983). Typical children may show elements of each style to varying degrees in their language development, and alternate at different points along the continuum between primarily Gestalt and primarily analytic processing (Peters 1977, 1980; Prizant 1983).

Krashen and Scarcella (1978) also identified two types of linguistic patterns, prefabricated routines and prefabricated patterns, as the primary strategies of Gestalt-style language acquisition for typical first and second language learners. Prefabricated routines refer to memorized whole utterances or phrases which a speaker may use without any knowledge of their internal structure. Prefabricated patterns refer to partly creative and partly memorized wholes, such as memorized sentence frames with an open slot for a phrase (e.g. "I want _____"; "This is a _____"). Prefabricated routines and prefabricated patterns appear to resemble

---

1   That is, the means to break down the field and/or pattern of language form into separate language components.

delayed echolalia and mitigated delayed echolalia, respectively (Prizant 1983).

Researchers who study Gestalt styles and Gestalt language forms in typical children acquiring language consider such linguistic patterns to be important, if not essential, to language acquisition and social interactive growth. Use of Gestalt forms of language acquisition, such as formulaic utterances, unanalyzed chunks, and prefabricated routines, provide children with a framework for developing more complex communicative skills. These findings can be applied to investigations of language acquisition in children with ASD and used to understand characteristics and deficits in autistic children's communicative behaviors.

Echolalic speech is mostly comprised of unanalyzed units of speech. As noted earlier, the language patterns of immediate echolalia and delayed echolalia and interactive inflexibility[2] are the most striking and prevalent features of communication of verbal autistic children. Each of these characteristics can be better understood as manifestations of Gestalt processing. A child with ASD who demonstrates immediate echolalia seems to be treating each repeated utterance as a unit, with a lack of appreciation of its internal constituent structure (Fay 1973; Prizant 1983). Even if the child demonstrates some comprehension of an utterance he or she echoes, such understanding is extremely limited (Prizant and Duchan 1981). The child's major strategy seems to be repeating utterances that are beyond his or her processing capacities, even though parts of the utterance may be recognized. This strategy is best achieved by a reproduction of the whole acoustic form, or the last section of a form, depending upon short-term memory limitations. The reproduction of the (whole) speech pattern has been associated with Gestalt or holistic modes of language processing (Prizant 1983).

Delayed echolalia is another good example of Gestalt processing because it seems to be an effort to bring forth whole forms that were heard previously in similar situations (Prizant 1983; Prizant *et al.* 1997). Therefore, delayed echoic patterns may be manifestations of Gestalt processing at both situational (i.e. context) and linguistic levels (Lord and Paul 1997; Prizant 1983). Children with ASD may produce multiword utterances as whole units, with little if any knowledge or understanding of the internal structure. After that, children may produce such unanalyzed units as a partial fulfillment for a situational cue or context, in which

---

2   An inflexibility when the child interacts with others. It is present in the child's social
     behaviors, emotional expression and communicative gestures, and language.

a child attempts to replicate a previous situation. Utterances in delayed echolalia might not refer to prior events, but might be a reproduction of portions or elements of the prior contexts that were retained in episodic memory (Prizant 1983).

In addition to patterns of immediate and delayed echolalia, inflexibility in social interactive patterns (i.e. adherence to routines, stereotypic conversational openers, or incessant questioning) also provides evidence for Gestalt processing in children with ASD (Prizant 1983). Verbal children with ASD may acquire knowledge of the structure of social interactions (e.g. "It is time to go"), but they demonstrate incompetence in handling the subtle adjustments and modifications necessary for an efficient exchange of information (e.g. "It is time to say goodbye"). Such observations suggest that children with ASD may be preoccupied with the predictability of the structure of interactive exchanges or its external framework (i.e. pattern), rather than with its internal content (i.e. the information shared). Prizant (1983) claimed that these rigid communicative or interactive patterns might be caused by an extreme form of Gestalt processing.

Gestalt language acquisition in children with ASD has been explained by the perception and production of patterns in their speech. Speech and language patterns of autistic children are characterized by repetition of unanalyzed forms that may be non-communicative or may be used as a means to express communicative intent. Such expressive patterns in autism may reflect Gestalt language acquisition, thus indicating an inability to analyze or segment others' utterances and recognize their internal structure (i.e. semantic-syntactic processing). Because some people with autism appear to be limited to an extreme style of Gestalt processing, the process of language acquisition, even for higher functioning autistic children, is truly challenging. Furthermore, those who may remain primarily echolalic might not move along the continuum toward an analytic processing of language due to their cognitive limitations (Prizant 1983).

Utilization of Gestalt principles in the development of functional speech

Greater perceptual and cognitive development in ASD probably allows some movement from a period of primarily Gestalt processing toward an analytic approach in language acquisition (Lord and Paul 1997; Prizant 1983). Defining this developmental process is necessary for enhancing language acquisition and speech production for children with ASD. How does the reproduction of memorized multiword units (i.e. echolalia) become the creative and generative linguistic process typically associated with the spontaneous production of multiword utterances? Prizant (1983) proposes a four-stage process of language acquisition from echolalia to spontaneous language. The four stages were designed from Prizant's observations of sequential language development in children with ASD who demonstrate echolalia. Prizant *et al.* (1997) suggested the appropriate interventions for language acquisition according to the proposed four stages of language acquisition.

The four-stage process is best understood as continuous, without clear points of delineation (Prizant 1983). In the first stage, utterances are predominantly echolalic and may fulfill a conversational "turn-taking," while other utterances may be produced for a self-stimulatory effect. According to Prizant, most accounts of speech in this early stage show little evidence of comprehension or communicative functions. The language enhancement strategies in the first stage might include: modifying situations or contexts in which echolalia or UVB are found to be correlated; simplifying language input; and varying interaction styles. At the end of the first stage, echolalia may represent a transitional phase to more conventional communication (Prizant *et al.* 1997).

In the second stage, a child's growth of general knowledge and relationships within the environment may exceed linguistic growth, and language remains predominantly echolalic (Prizant 1983). Due to cognitive growth and experiences in social interaction, a greater variety of functions will be served by echolalia. A child might attempt to express intentions and to comment on relationships within the environment by using echolalia. In addition, echolalia may serve as a means of behavioral self-regulation and as a rehearsal strategy. Toward the end of the second stage, a child might also apply particular strategies to break down echolalic utterances and acquire one- and two-word utterances. These strategies allow for an increased understanding of the constituent structure of utterances (i.e. speech patterns) and of the semantic relationships encoded in the utterances. Introduction of conventional, non-speech augmentative communicative means, such as pictures, gestures, or signs, may be an important strategy at this time (Prizant *et al.* 1997).

The third stage is mainly characterized by increasing flexibility in language structure, and simultaneous use of both spontaneous and echolalic utterances. This stage includes a period in which similar communicative functions are served by spontaneous and echolalic utterances, followed by a decrease in echolalia with a concomitant increase in spontaneous speech.

As pure echolalic speech decreases, speech repetition becomes more flexible and less rigidly produced. In other words, echolalia becomes mitigated with increased modifications and with decreased exact reproductions.

In this third stage, a child might acquire linguistic forms governed by knowledge of early semantic and syntactic rules. A further segmentation or combination of echolalic utterances also occurs, which may be part of the process of acquiring more spontaneous forms of speech patterns. More creative speech patterns begin to emerge as well. Therefore, modeling language in a context of active involvement and in synchrony with relevant action patterns is a powerful teaching strategy. Replacing pure echolalia with more conventional means to communicate, such as intraverbal communication or verbal cueing,[3] could be an effective strategy at this stage.

In the final stage of language acquisition, more spontaneous and flexible language is demonstrated, thus reflecting an increasing knowledge of semantic-syntactic and morphological rules. A more rule-governed and generative linguistic system might be developed in the final stage. Echolalia no longer serves primary communicative functions, because the child has become capable of operating the language system. As a result, the child is able to process language and regulate communication. Communicative functions are now served primarily by creative, spontaneous utterances. In this stage, it is essential that the language environment includes stimuli that are relevant and meaningful in context. Decision making and choice making in daily activities might provide a motivating context for the child to learn to use more conventional forms of verbal behavior with clear consequences (Prizant *et al.* 1997).

In conclusion, echolalic speech can be used to acquire functional language in children with ASD. According to Prizant's four-stage developmental process of language acquisition, echolalia is the starting point, and therefore should be encouraged at the first stage. At the second stage, the link between echolalic response and other experiences and stimuli should be established. At the third stage, echolalia needs to be shaped by modification of speech patterns toward more flexible and spontaneous speech. Certain behavior modification strategies such as modeling, cueing, and reinforcement might be helpful in this stage. At the final stage, functional and spontaneous use of language is accomplished.

---

3   Intraverbal communication is a type of expressive language where a word or phrase called verbal cueing evokes another word or phrase, but the two are not identical. It resembles word association, such as the tendency to say "mouse" when someone says "Mickey."

Eventual segmentation of Gestalt forms and echolalic speech patterns with rule induction[4] allow for greater creativity and generativity in the speech production of children with ASD (Prizant 1983; Prizant *et al.* 1997). Expansion and reduction of Gestalt forms of speech patterns have been shown to be effective strategies in helping children with ASD to produce more functional, rule-governed utterances (Scherer and Olswang 1989; Sundberg and Partington 1998). Modifying UVB or echolalia and teaching intraverbal behaviors will enhance speech development in children with ASD (Prizant *et al.* 1997; Sundberg and Partington 1998). Gestalt-style language acquisition, including pattern perception, anticipation, and planning of speech production, may eventually elicit spontaneous speech.

A major achievement in language development for children with ASD is movement from single-unit communication to a combination of units, reflecting knowledge of early semantic-syntactic relationships. This goal may be approached through clear modeling of multiword utterances, in natural as well as contrived contexts, and based on both developmental and functional needs. Therefore, expansion of single-unit language in contrived and naturalistic learning settings is the necessary process in speech development for children with ASD (Paul and Sutherland 2005; Prizant and Wetherby 2005; Prizant *et al.* 1997).

Many children with ASD demonstrate progressive changes in their echolalic utterances, leading to the emergence of some degree of more creative, rule-governed linguistic behavior (Prizant *et al.* 1997). Echolalia can eventually serve a variety of cognitive and social-communicative functions and may become the vehicle by which children with ASD acquire more conventional language forms (Lord and Paul 1997; Prizant *et al.* 1997). Research has indicated that UVB, including echolalia, are more likely to occur in some situational and communicative contexts than in others (Prizant 1983; Prizant and Duchan 1981; Rydell and Mirenda 1991). It is common for echolalia to be produced initially with limited communicative intent and used later with increased intention. Due to the Gestalt style of language acquisition in ASD, it is possible that these children will rely on echolalia and repetition of speech in interacting with others.

---

4   The segmentation of Gestalt forms and echolalic speech patterns is a process of breaking down the whole form or creating more chunks of the whole form into more simplified forms/ patterns.

As noted earlier, some forms of echolalia are highly unconventional, and therefore may be barriers to effective communication. Other forms, however, are clearly produced with intent and will be more recognizable because of their greater conventionality and relevance to the communicative context. In order to use echolalia in enhancing speech and language development, intervention should involve appropriate contexts containing communicative exchanges and activities of high motivation and interest. Furthermore, interventions or activities must be engaged in functional language use, cognitive learning, and independence (Prizant *et al.* 1997).

3

Music Perception and Speech and Language Perception

Music perception

Gestalt laws of music perception

Music is composed of many separate yet interconnected components such as pitch, melody, rhythm, harmony, form, timbre, and dynamics. These elements are typically arranged in patterns and perceived as "music." These musical patterns are organized in such a way as to bring anticipation of incoming patterns over a temporal order (Berger 2002). Musical pattern perception is commonly ruled by Gestalt laws of perception (Radocy and Boyle 2003). Gestalt psychology emphasizes the importance of figure-ground relationships in perceptual pattern organization. Gestalt psychologists have proposed a number of organizational principles including proximity, similarity, common direction, simplicity, and closure (Eysenck 2001). The law of proximity states that objects that are close to one another tend to be grouped together. Similarity involves the grouping of objects that share common attributes. A common direction results when either visual or aural objects appear to have the same motion trajectory. Simplicity (i.e. good continuation) means that perceptual organization will always be as good as prevailing conditions allow, and closure involves the perceptual completion of an object that is physically incomplete. These laws assist in the process of recognizing the most important sensory events and abstracting them perceptually from a less significant background of activity.

Similar perceptual processes are at work when perceiving organized patterns in music (Eysenck 2001; Lipscomb 1996; Radocy and Boyle 2003). Essentially, the Gestalt perceptual laws as applied to melodic perception suggest that listeners are likely to perceive musical tones close together in time and auditory space as a melodic unit (i.e. proximity). The listeners tend to perceive similar, repeated tones as a unit (i.e. similarity), and hear a melodic sequence as moving in a common direction toward completion (i.e. common direction) based on what they heard previously. In addition, listeners are likely to perceive and organize the Gestalt, the melodic contour or pattern, in its simplest form (i.e. simplicity) (Radocy and Boyle 2003).

Musical patterns are necessary for cortical perception (Berger 2002). As soon as information is perceived as structured and organized musical patterns, which the brain prefers to process rather than random items, the brain begins activation in the higher channels of cognition. Berger (2002) states that children with ASD might also utilize this perceptual-pattern organization in processing musical sounds.

Grouping: the perceptual segmentations of musical sounds

Grouping refers to the perception of boundaries, with elements between boundaries clustering together to form a temporal unit. In music, grouping is the perceptual clustering of musical tones into chunks larger than single tones but smaller than the entire melody. Music perception relies on perceptual grouping (Patel 2008). This suggests that perceptual grouping enables the mental chunking process of musical sounds. Grouping of musical sounds is conceived as hierarchical, with lower level groups placed within higher level ones. The hierarchies (i.e. different level groups) in musical sounds are perceived as categories in music. Durations in musical rhythms, harmonic structures (i.e. chord progressions), intervals (i.e. pitch relationship), melodies, and musical forms are perceived in terms of categories. Interestingly, many empirical studies found that grouping, the hierarchical and categorical perception, plays a prominent role in the study of rhythm, prosody (intonation in speech), and syntax in speech (Patel 2008).

Similarities between music and speech and language perception

Common perceptual mechanisms in music and speech and language

Perception of musical elements is similar in many ways to the perception of speech and language information. Patel (2008) stated in his book titled *Music, Language and the Brain* that, from the perspective of cognitive neuroscience, both music and language systems depend on mental framework-perceived (learned) sound categories. In other words, music and language share mechanisms for sound category perception and learning to a very important degree.

Rhythm perception is similar to perception of numbers in a metric organization (i.e. counting) (Clarke 1987; Radocy and Boyle 2003; Sloboda 1985). A number of research studies confirm the role of rhythmic predictability in speech perception (Patel 2008). In particular, rhythm plays an important role in anticipating stress location in syllables, producing accents segmenting connected speech. Patterns of timing and accent in musical rhythm are a focus of rhythm in language. In addition, timbre or dynamic perception is directly involved in the perception of intensity, quantity, or quality.

Some researchers believe that intonation in music is synonymous with speech melody (Bolinger 1985); this suggests a strong connection between melody perception and perception of linguistic intonation. Melodic contour perception is important in both music and speech. It is possible that the processing of melodic contour in the two domains is mediated by common cognitive and neural mechanisms. Trehub and Trainor (1993) indicated that pitch-contour processes in music perception and prosodic processes in speech require a common auditory perceptual strategy.[1] The sequential patterns of ups and downs in a melody define its pitch contour, and a pitch contour with its temporal patterns defines a melodic contour. The melodic contour relates to the pitch pattern of the spoken phrases (Patel 2008).

Melodic contour also plays an important role in the immediate memory of the phrases (Patel 2008). Memory of musical elements such as memory of melody contour or rhythm pattern is based on the perceptual organization of sequential structure. Thus, it is similar to learning speech or to memory of events (Radocy and Boyle 2003). Music perception follows the same principles of general perceptual organization, such as pattern recognition and grouping information into categorical units. The mechanism of music perception is similar to the perceptional and cognitive mechanism of speech and language information (Radocy and Boyle 2003; Thaut 2005). The

---

1   Pitch contour refers to the process of creating particular patterns of ascending and descending pitches in a melody's sequence of perceived tones. The process requires the perception of the fixed pitches in music and it is a categorical nature of pitch perception. Some analogies between linguistic and musical structures can be found; prosody refers to the speech-sound classes of language which include the particular patterns of ascending and descending pitches in a sequence of speech sound. Prosody reflects a range of sounds along a pitch continuum, and is actually perceived as a given sound unit. Similarly, the perception prosody might use fixed pitches in speech sound, and is perceived categorically.

similarities between music and speech and language suggest a link between the two domains in terms of their evolution and development.

McMullen and Saffran (2004) explain that both music and language are organized temporally, with pattern structures unfolding in time. Furthermore, both speech and music reach the perceptual system as frequency spectra arrayed as pitches, which are generated from a finite set of sounds (notes or phonemes), selected from a larger possible set of sounds. These sounds are organized into discrete categories which facilitate recalling and representation of the sounds. In other words, auditory events in both language and music domains are subject to the process of categorical pattern perception (McMullen and Saffran 2004).

General auditory processing mechanisms responsible for pattern analysis are involved in the perception of both speech and music. The vast stores of knowledge pertaining to these separate domains, however, may be stored in separate places in the brain (Patel 2003). Basic similarities between speech and music learning mechanisms would be expected. McMullen and Saffran (2004) reported that brain mapping research data overwhelmingly support separate cortical regions sub-serving some aspects of musical and linguistic processing in adults. Young children may bring some of the same skills to bear on learning in each domain. The brains of young children are quite plastic and show a remarkable ability to reorganize auditory events, which suggests that early experience or training has a profound effect on the cortical and perceptual organization of auditory stimuli (McMullen and Saffran 2004).

A large body of research literature regarding music and language supports the idea that their roots are indistinguishable. In particular, the early perception of sound seems to involve common processes across music and language (Hafteck 1997; McMullen and Saffran 2004; Michel and Jones 1992). There is evidence of grouping processes such as repeating the same utterance in infancy for both music and language. Both musical and spoken phrases are perceptual units for infants, and their perception is based on larger units such as pitch contour and rhythmic structure (Hafteck 1997). This perceptual phenomenon is found in egocentric speech and spontaneous songs of infants. Furthermore, pitch-contour processing is an important perceptual organizational device for infants not only for processing musical sequences, but also for speech sequences, especially the prosodic aspects of speech (Hafteck 1997; Trehub and Trainor 1993).

From the early perception of sounds to the emergence of singing and speech, a close relationship between music and language development is evident. During the early stages of development, when music and speech are highly integrated, the closer link between the two domains should be encouraged (Hafteck 1997). From the perspective of young listeners, who must learn about each system of music and speech before discovering its communicative intent, the similarities between music and speech perceptions may be heightened. Due to the similarities, children might learn how to speak and sing in close tandem; furthermore, music can incorporate singing and speech in a very structurally cohesive way (Thaut 2005).

Shared mechanisms in the perception of musical and linguistic sounds mean that listeners might develop a mental framework that allows learning of both music and speech. If there are shared mechanisms for learning the sound of speech and music, an individual's ability to perceive sounds in one domain should have some predictive power with regard to perception of sounds in the other domain. Research on children and adults supports this prediction through the findings that pitch-related musical abilities predict phonological skills in speech (Patel 2008). Furthermore, if there are common mechanisms that the brain uses to convert sound waves into discrete sound categories in speech and music, then it is conceivable that perceptually exercising these mechanisms with sounds from one domain could enhance the ability of these mechanisms to acquire sound categories in the other domain.

Neuro-anatomical commonalities between music and speech perception

Many experimental investigations have tested the idea that exposure to music benefits speech and language due to the perceptual similarities (Schön, Magne and Besson 2004). One way to explore the speech–music link is to examine the neuro-anatomical relationship between the two domains. Patients have been tested with either speech and language deficits or music perception deficits following brain damage in order to find the common cortical regions or neural pathways involved in both music and speech. The development of brain-imaging techniques offers new possibilities for testing the hypothesis that music influences other cognitive domains including speech and language. The results of these neuro-anatomical studies might provide more conclusive answers for the link between music and speech.

Patel *et al.* (1998) examined the relationship between the perceptual processing of melodic and rhythmic patterns in speech and music. They tested the prosodic and musical discrimination abilities of two amusic[2] patients who had music perception deficits secondary to bilateral brain damage. Results revealed parallel perceptual processes between linguistic prosody and musical structure in the two patients. Patel *et al.* (1998) found preservation of both prosodic and musical discrimination abilities in one amusic patient, and impairments of both abilities in the other amusic patient. This result indicates that perception of speech prosody and melodic contour share common cognitive and neural resources, as does the perception of rhythmic patterns in speech and music (Patel *et al.* 1998). In both amusic patients, the level of performance was similar across domains, suggesting that they shared the same neural resources and structures for prosody and music. Patel *et al.* (1998) indicate that prosody in speech and music may overlap in the processes used to maintain the auditory patterns in working memory.

A case study of an aphasic patient with brain damage was conducted in order to explore the perception and memory of texts and melodies in songs (Peretz *et al.* 2004). The patient had a severe speech disorder, marked by phonemic errors and stuttering, without a concomitant musical production disorder. The patient was instructed to repeat song lines in a sung version (with words), a "la, la, la" version (singing a melody without words), and a spoken version. The performance of the melody version was significantly higher than the performance of the spoken version (i.e. text), and singing did not help the patient's articulation of syllables. In addition, the characteristics of the errors were similar in the singing and speaking versions. The impairment in speech, such as the disruption of speech planning procedures, affected both speaking and singing in a similar manner. Speech disruption, however, left melodic production intact. The speech route was distinct from the spared melodic route. Peretz *et al.* (2004) concluded that verbal production, whether it was sung or spoken, was mediated by the same impaired language output system. The neural pathway of speech production, however, was distinct from the spared pathway of melody production (Peretz *et al.* 2004).

Brown *et al.* (2004) examined the activation of the cortical system using brain-imaging while amateur musicians sang repetitions of novel melodies, sang harmonization with novel melodies, or vocalized monotonically. Major blood flow increased in the primary and secondary auditory cortex, primary motor cortex, frontal operculum, supplementary motor

---

2   Amusia means "without music," referring to a form of aphasia characterized by an inability to produce or recognize music.

area, insula, posterior cerebellum, and basal ganglia during monotonic vocalization and melody repetition. Melody repetition and harmonization produced patterns of cortical activation very similar to each other; however, harmonization, as compared to the results for melody repetition, showed more intense activations in the same areas (Brown *et al.* 2004).

The results also revealed a strong overlap in cortical activation during the monotonic vocalization, melody repetition, and harmonization tasks. This overlapping brain activation suggests that participants perceived monotonic vocalization as a musical task, despite the use of a single pitch (Brown *et al.* 2004). Vocalization with a steady beat might be perceived as a simple form of music. This antiphonal, monotonic vocalization task should be seen as a model of some of the most important (cardinal) features of music (Brown *et al.* 2004). The results also revealed that the melody repetition and harmonization tasks required the activation of a part of the tertiary auditory cortex which is specialized for higher level pitch processing and the storage of pitch information in working memory.

Brown *et al.* (2004) proposed the existence of a cortical system that is specialized for imitative auditory behavior, including antiphonal imitation, and that such a system would be a foundation for audio-vocal matching functions, such as song and speech. Both music and speech development in children are based on a process of imitating adult role models during critical periods in brain development. The frontal operculum in Broca's area could be the system of antiphonal imitation and the antiphonal production of song, since the system involves audio-vocal matching for both pitch and rhythm. Therefore, Broca's area might process pitch and rhythm information in music, and transfer the information into motor aspects of vocalization. Brown *et al.* (2004) conclude that the imitative function of Broca's area is directly involved in the imitative audio-vocal processes underlying music and speech. They further suggest that singing is mediated by a vocalization system based on antiphonal imitation in the frontal operculum of Broca's area (Brown *et al.* 2004).

More recently, in order to examine a direct neuro-anatomical link between music and language, parallel generational tasks for melody and speech were compared using positron emission tomography (Brown, Martinez and Parsons 2006). Ten right-handed amateur musicians were asked to vocally improvise melodies or sentences, while PET scans were performed to measure cortical activations while performing the improvisational tasks. The overall results of the study suggest that common, parallel, and distinctive neural mechanisms for music and language might exist (Brown *et al.* 2006). The results indicate that a striking overlap exists in the brain activations between music and speech conditions (Brown *et al.* 2006). The overlapping activations were found in the primary auditory cortex, sub-cortical auditory system, and motor cortex underlying vocalization. This indicates that both music and language tasks require common perceptual processing of auditory stimuli and share neural resources for the control of phonation and articulation during singing and speaking.

The parallel activations for music and speech were found in the secondary auditory cortex that is involved in the perceptual processing of complex sound patterns, and in Broca's area where vocal production and syntax processing are generated (Brown *et al.* 2006). The secondary auditory cortex is an interface area for organizing patterns of sounds and interpreting the phonology of complex sounds and then transmitting it to areas supporting the semantics of words and phrases. A parallel activation in the secondary auditory cortex was found while processing pitch, interval, and scale structure in a melody generation task. In addition, Broca's area was activated by the vocal production of melody and the sequential ordering of music which is processed in a similar manner to language syntax (Brown *et al.* 2006). The regions of parallel activation might share the common decoding or encoding system for music and language, or the neural system might have an "adaptive coding" capacity to process different types of information (i.e. music or language).

The distinct, non-overlapping, domain-specific activations in extra temporal areas were observed for the melody and sentence generation tasks. Brown *et al.* (2006) indicate that these distinctive cortical activations might result from task operation-related differences, particularly different informational content (i.e. semantics). Collectively, melody and sentence generating tasks share neural processing in the primary auditory cortex and primary motor cortex in this PET study. Parallel representations for phonological processing and sound sequences in speech and music were observed in the secondary auditory cortex and in Broca's area. Finally, domain-specific and non-overlapping representations for distinctive functions in music and language were also found (Brown *et al.* 2006).

In summary, researchers have found neuro-anatomical structures that are involved in both music and speech perception and production. Broca's area, the primary and secondary auditory cortices (i.e. bilateral temporal and right inferior frontal lobe), and the primary motor cortex are the regions involved in processing both music and speech, particularly prosody in speech (Brown *et al.* 2004, 2006; Patel *et al.* 1998). Even though the neural pathways are not identical between the production of music and speech, similar patterns of cortical activation have been observed in the perception and production of music and speech.

4

Perception and Production of Music and Speech in Children with ASD

Music has been used for ASD treatment for decades because of the beneficial effects of musical stimuli and the positive musical responses in children with ASD. Since 1965, music therapy literature has reported the positive effects of musical activities on cognitive, social, and sensory development for children with ASD. A few music therapy studies have focused on the positive effect of music on communication and language improvement. This chapter reviews research literature regarding music perception and production in children with ASD and the link between music and speech production.

Perception of music in children with ASD

As discussed earlier, children with ASD may have abnormal auditory-cortical activation that causes a dysfunction of specific temporal regions which specialize in the processing of spoken words and the integration of complex sounds (Boddaert *et al.* 2004). Nevertheless, the majority of children with ASD show an intact ability to perceive and produce complex sounds, including musical sounds (Schuler 1995; Tager-Flusberg 1997). A distinct sensitivity and attention to music has been frequently mentioned in the literature on children with ASD (Thaut 1999). Some ASD children respond favorably and appropriately to musical sounds (Thaut 1999). Children with ASD are able to perceive and produce well-organized musical patterns, such as melodic and rhythmic patterns. This section reviews the music literature regarding the music behaviors of children with ASD, including their perception and production of music.

Thaut (1987) investigated the perceptual preferences of children with autism by comparing their responses to musical and visual stimuli. Each child was given the choice of watching picture-slides or listening to music. Children with autism showed a slight preference for the musical stimulus, and stayed significantly longer in the music than in the visual condition. By contrast, children matched by chronological age and developmental age preferred the visual stimulus over the music. Most children with autism showed strong motor reactions, such as jumping up and down in the chair, body rocking, and swinging the torso, whenever the music was playing (Thaut 1987). There is a marked difference in preference and response to music between children with autism and typical children. Children with autism have a perceptual preference for and an intact capacity to perceive auditory musical stimuli. In spite of their developmental deficits, children with autism are able to perceive musical sounds in a meaningful way. Moreover, the musical preference and sensitivity of autistic children can be positively transferred to their non-musical behaviors by activating the common perceptual mechanisms (Thaut 1987).

Children with ASD who have affective and interpersonal deficits can perceive affect in music (Heaton, Hermelin and Pring 1999). Children with and without ASD were asked to identify the affective patterns in musical melodies by matching musical mode (i.e. major or minor key) with happy and sad faces. The results showed that children with and without ASD did not differ in their ability to identify the affective patterns in major and minor musical modes. In spite of their affective and interpersonal deficits, children with ASD showed no deficit in processing affective patterns in musical stimuli. Heaton *et al.* (1999) concluded that children with ASD could recognize emotional expression in music at a simple level, and that they might have an intact perception of melody patterns in music, such as a key or melodic mode. Furthermore, they appear to have an intact perceptual ability to connect the musical pattern with a corresponding affective pattern.

In summary, the perception of musical stimuli is intact in some children with ASD, and that they often have a perceptual preference for music. Musical stimuli are commonly organized and perceived by patterns, and this musical pattern perception is observed in children with ASD (Heaton *et al.* 1999; Lim 2009, 2010; Orr, Myles and Carlson 1998). Pattern perception is also the primary mechanism for speech and language in children with ASD. In particular, language development in children with ASD is heavily influenced by their capacity for pattern perception and production (Lim 2010; Prizant

1983; Prizant *et al.* 1997). Thus, it is suggested that pattern perception is the common phenomenon in children with ASD for processing both music and speech (Berger 2002; Thaut 2005).

Pattern perception of music and speech in children with ASD

Pattern perception

Previous research has explored the commonalities in pattern processing and organization for both language and music. Therefore, it is worthwhile to examine how the perception and production of musical elements relates to the perception and production of the corresponding patterns in language. In addition, how children with ASD perceive and produce the primary elements or patterns in both music and speech needs to be explored. As in music, in language the presence of patterns is very evident. Every word, when divided into its syllabic rhythm, displays patterns. The functions of patterns in speech and language can be found in musical patterns.

Rhythmic patterns

In music, rhythm provides the temporal ordering of sounds and is perceived as a temporal figure based on the beat patterns. Rhythmic patterns are organized by grouping and perceived as a unit. In addition, rhythmic patterns have constancy and a repetitive nature. The continuity and perseverative nature of rhythm provides the perceptual elements that ultimately facilitate focused cortical activation, since the brain attends to the repetitive nature of the pulse interacting with rhythmic patterns (Berger 2002; Thaut 2005). Rhythm is considered one of the most important elements in the learning of spoken language. The temporal pattern in language embellishes and causes the anticipation of the following pattern (Barrett 1999; Peters 1983). Berger (2002) suggests that nonverbal children with autism tend to be more attentive and motivated to imitate and learn word sounds that are broken down into rhythmically patterned syllables, spoken, clapped, and/or sung. A simple verbal phrase repeated to a rhythmic pattern might sustain the children's attention and interest in the verbal input and increase their anticipation of the following phrase.

Pitch, melodic contour, and prosody

In music, pitch is a psychological property of tones that is perceived categorically (e.g. C, D#, G). Frequency, the physiological property of tone, produces certain patterns of neural excitation in the higher auditory pathway. Listeners tend to perceive these patterns and organize them into a certain category (Patel 2008; Radocy and Boyle 2003). Perceived patterns are stored and recalled as pitch memory. Organized patterns of different pitches constitute a melody in music, as well as prosody of speech.

Perception of melody is based on melodic contour, which is the overall shape or particular pattern of pitch movements. Melodic contour strengthened by rhythm is commonly perceived as a Gestalt or whole figure. Therefore, melody perception follows the principles of Gestalt perceptual organization (Lipscomb 1996; Radocy and Boyle 2003). In the perception of melody, hierarchical orders of melodic contour are based on the temporal structure. In other words, the rhythmic pattern is a necessary perceptual unit for melody perception. Melodic patterns or contours, such as wide sweeps and leaps from low to high pitches (e.g. "Twinkle, twinkle, little star"), or scale-wise melodies (e.g. "Mary had a little lamb"), create different physiological and psychological states of anticipation in listeners (Berger 2002; Radocy and Boyle 2003). Therefore, melodic songs can stimulate a center in the brain that analyzes different sequences of pitch and processes the melodic pattern, such as Broca's area. Melodic contour might facilitate the center to intone the prosody of letters or words in songs, and then eventually to lead to proper speech production.

The ability to analyze auditory information accurately in a melodic pattern is of vital importance in learning speech prosody. Prosody refers to the variation of tones used when speaking (i.e. intonation or pitch) and vocal stress, which is the relative emphasis given to certain syllables in a word (McCann and Peppe 2003). The functions of prosody are to provide an indication of the speech affect and speaker's intention. Many children with ASD lack speech affect or prosody (Tager-Flusberg 1997). They are, however, able to imitate melodic patterns in songs and produce prosody in musical speech (Edgerton 1994; Wigram 2000). Children with ASD might be able to express their emotions through musical melodies, and furthermore to produce prosodic vocal self-expression through melodic patterns.

Dynamics

In music, perception of sound intensity occurs via patterns of energy, resonance, and level of auditory stimulation through the variance of volume (Berger 2002; Radocy and Boyle 2003). A listener is immediately engaged by dynamic nuances, because other musical elements such as melody or rhythm are emphasized by dynamics. Patterns of musical dynamics such as loud, soft, and gradual increases and decreases of volume contribute to the emotional content of music. In particular, dynamics indicate intention and emotion of a musical passage (i.e. musical prosody). Music dynamics parallel human dynamics in terms of moods, levels of excitability, and physical and psychological states (Berger 2002; Thaut 2005). The ability to perceive and produce dynamics in music can be used in the perception and production of the dynamics of speech which also indicate the urgency and level of the emotional state.

In individuals with ASD, it is not unusual to find either very few dynamics in their playing of musical instruments or predominantly loud mono-dynamic pounding. By contrast, some musical expressions by children with ASD display erratic dynamic changes, such as overall soft playing, except for a sudden loud attack. These musical displays are possibly due to impairments in expression of inner states and reciprocal social interaction.

Form and structure

Musical form is another type of auditory pattern. Since musical form ultimately shapes the musical pattern development and limits the size of the pattern presentation, it elicits the anticipation of structural closure. Musical form evokes cognitive processes for planning and organizing (Berger 2002). Perception of musical form is based on perceiving the repetition of a combination of musical elements and anticipating the upcoming patterns within a given time frame.

Perception of musical form might be related to the semantic and pragmatic aspects of language. Such aspects as how a tune begins, where it goes next, how long it should continue, how it can conclude, and how many repetitions would be enough are evident in both musical and speech form. According to Berger (2002), attention is actually a state of anticipation. The brain waits and attends to information by remaining in a holding pattern until some resolution allows the processing to conclude.

This particular perceptual process can be applied to semantic and pragmatic language ability.

Linguistic form and sentence structure have been used in developing language teaching methods for children with language impairments and ASD (Sundberg and Partington 1998). Once children understand a particular form or sentence structure, they tend to perceive new elements (e.g. vocabulary words) easily within this structure (Sundberg and Partington 1998). Repetitive learning is needed to acquire a particular language pattern, and eventually leads to linguistic memory.

In conclusion, the perception of music parallels the perception of language, and these processes appear to be intact in children with ASD. Both musical stimuli and language stimuli are perceived as patterns in the sensory channels of children with ASD. Research has shown that children with ASD perceive and produce speech-sounds or words in musical songs in the same way that typical children do, in spite of their dysfunction in auditory areas (Edgerton 1994; Wigram 2000; Wimpory and Nash 1999). Children with ASD also appear to have intact neuro-anatomical regions for processing speech sounds, as well as musical elements, including melody, rhythm, and structure in songs. Musical patterns may stimulate and activate intact neural processes for auditory information (Berger 2002; Heaton *et al.* 1999; Thaut 1988).

Musical perception and production in children with ASD

Research has indicated that children with ASD recognize and perceive patterns in music (Berger 2002; Heaton *et al.* 1999; Lim 2010; Orr *et al.* 1998; Thaut 1987). Analysis of the literature indicates that the mechanism of musical behaviors in children with ASD is based on pattern perception and production. If children with ASD have an intact ability to perceive musical patterns, it is worthwhile to explore their capacity to produce well-organized musical patterns, such as melodic and rhythmic patterns.

Musical behavior in children with ASD

Thaut (1988) analyzed improvised musical tone sequences produced by three groups of children: with autism, without autism, and with intellectual disabilities. The children were asked to play a xylophone arranged in a pentatonic scale, and were allowed to continue playing until they came to a natural ending. The produced musical tone sequences were then analyzed according to the following five criteria: rhythm, restriction, complexity, rule adherence of melodic subunits, and originality. Rhythm indicated the imposition of and adherence to temporal order, and restriction indicated the use of available musical elements. Complexity indicated the generation of recurring melodic patterns, rule adherence of melodic subunits indicated the application of melodic patterns to the total sound sequences, and originality indicated the production of original melodic patterns.

The results suggested that children with autism scored significantly higher than children with intellectual disabilities in terms of rhythm, restriction, originality, and total performance score. No significant differences were found between typical children and children with autism in terms of rhythm, restriction, total performance score, or originality. These findings indicate that the overall performance of children with autism was not significantly inferior to typical children. Among the three groups of children, children with autism achieved the highest mean score on the restriction scale, and the lowest mean score on the complexity scale (Thaut 1988).

The rhythmic scores by children with autism might reflect a tendency to adhere rigidly to temporal rules. Their high scores for restriction showed that children with autism perceive and explore the available musical material just as typically developing children do. In terms of complexity and rule adherence, the tone sequences of children with autism showed some abnormal features, resembling the performance of children with intellectual disabilities, by being relatively short and repetitive. The low performance on complexity and rule adherence of children with autism suggest that they might have difficulty organizing and retaining complex temporal sequences. In summary, the results indicate that some children with autism are able to produce musical tone sequences containing melodic and rhythmic patterns. Moreover, musical pattern production in children with autism appeared to be not much different from that of typically developing children.

The communicative and interactive behaviors of children with autism are commonly presented through their musical behaviors. Eleven children with ASD were asked to improvise musical patterns on various musical instruments, including voice, piano, snare drum, and cymbal, in an interactive music therapy setting (Edgerton 1994). The children were able to match a fast basic beat to the experimenter's playing, simultaneously imitate the rhythm of a melodic motif, and participate in exchanging rhythmic patterns with the experimenter during improvisational instrument playing. A number of verbal, vocal, and instrumental behaviors were initiated by the children in an attempt to influence the experimenter's improvisation or musical behaviors. The analysis indicates that children with ASD are able to produce various rhythmic patterns, vocalize in a steady tempo, and match the tempo of their improvisation to the experimenter's varied tempo. In addition, they all produced vocal responses to varied pitches.

Edgerton (1994) found a significant positive correlation between the musical vocal behavior and the non-musical speech production: as musical vocal behaviors increased, non-musical speech production behaviors, such as verbal communication with gestures, also increased. Edgerton (1994) explained that communication through music might bypass the speech and language barriers of children with autism. Her study suggests that music improvisation might be effective at eliciting and increasing communicative behaviors in children with ASD within a musical setting (Edgerton 1994).

Children with ASD have certain behavioral characteristics, and some behaviors define the disorder. Children with autism also have certain characteristics in their musical behaviors. Edgerton (1994) found communicativeness and flexibility in musical instrument playing by children with ASD. By contrast, different results were found in a more recent study. Wigram (2000) described the musical behaviors and interactions of children with ASD in order to design a music therapy assessment tool for children with autism and communication disorders. According to Wigram's observation, classic rigidity was the main characteristic in musical instrument playing of children with autism. This musical behavior was observed in repetitive and unvarying rhythm pattern production, unchanging tempo, and lack of leading during the interactive playing with others. A restricted pattern producing style was presented through unvaried volume, tempo, and other musical elements (e.g. pitch range). Their musical playing was also considered to be systematic and methodical (Wigram 2000).

According to Wigram (2000), children with ASD produced perseverative and repetitive scale playing on the piano, xylophone, and metallophone, and made monotonous rhythm sequences on the guitar and the autoharp. In addition, children with ASD demonstrated a lack of skill or intuitive ability in turn-taking, sharing, anticipating, copying, reflecting, or empathic playing. These children also showed a lack of ability to respond to or share changes in tempo, rhythm, timbre, intensity, and many other elements of shared musical engagement. Children with ASD were, however, able to copy varied rhythm patterns and imitate the changes in scales on the keyboard. With repetitive experience and practice, children with ASD produced varied rhythm figures and more flexible tempi and dynamics (Wigram 2000).

These findings suggest that children with ASD produce musical patterns, although the patterns are restrictive. Furthermore, some children with autism perceive other people's musical patterns, and then change their own musical patterns accordingly. Restrictive and unrefined musical behaviors might be changed or corrected through imitating less restrictive and more refined patterns. Children with ASD might replace restrictive patterns with more varied and advanced musical patterns with appropriate training and practice.

Research has indicated that children with ASD have intact auditory areas that can process various patterns in sounds, including musical sounds and speech. The children's similar perceptual mechanisms in music and speech have been discussed. If children with autism can produce less restricted and more varied patterns by imitating other people's musical patterns, it is worthwhile to apply this learning process to the production of speech patterns. Children with ASD might produce more advanced speech patterns by imitating musical patterns in a song which contains such elements of the speech patterns as vocabulary words, rhythm pattern, prosody, and form. The perception and production of musical patterns might positively influence the perception and production of speech in children with ASD.

5

The Effect of Music on Speech and Language in Children with ASD

Analysis of the research findings in the effect of music stimuli on speech, language, and communication in children with ASD

A few researchers have explored the influence of music on speech and language skills in children with language impairments, including children with ASD. Hoskins (1988) investigated the relationship between sung and spoken versions of two standardized speech tests, and examined the effect of music on language abilities. Sixteen children with intellectual disabilities ranging in age from two to five years old took the Expressive One-Word Picture Vocabulary Test (EOWPVT: Gardner 1979) and the Peabody Picture Vocabulary Test (PPVT: Dunn and Dunn 1981) in its original form and in a modified sung version. In addition, three pre-recorded music subtests designed by Hoskins were used to determine participants' rhythm imitation, pitch imitation, and melodic imitation abilities. For each subtest, participants were asked to repeat the item immediately after hearing it. Participants attended ten weeks of music activities with an emphasis on increasing expressive language skills, including group singing (e.g. action songs) and antiphonal singing (Hoskins 1988).

The results of pre- and post-tests showed significant differences between each of the six pre-tests and post-tests. A statistically significant improvement in responses to the sung version of the PPVT was found in the pre- to post-test analysis. Hoskins (1988) indicated that the beneficial effect of antiphonal singing with picture cards might exist on the improvement of the melodic version of the language test. The sung version of the language test may have been more similar to the antiphonal singing in the music treatment, and this could indicate why significant improvement was found in the melodic version but not in the spoken version. The results also indicated a strong positive correlation between the spoken and sung versions of the PPVT. Pre- and post-tests of the spoken and sung versions of the PPVT were highly related, so that they could be said to measure the same attribute, and that no advantage exists for using one version over the other (Hoskins 1988). Children with ASD might perceive the auditory pattern equally well, whether it is in a sung version or in a spoken version. The positive effects for music in this study were largely attributed to an increased attention factor (Hoskins 1988).

Hoskins's study demonstrates how musical patterns integrate with speech patterns. The spoken version of a standard speech test was transformed into a musical form, a sung version of the same test. In addition, the sung version of the speech test measured speech and language ability in children with ASD. The results suggest that musical activities such as singing could be used to enhance scores on standardized language tests (Hoskins 1988).

More recently, Buday (1995) explored the use of music as a strategy to promote better short-term memory for manual signs in children with autism. Buday (1995) explained that many children with autism respond positively to music, and accounted for this effect in terms of attention to a regularly repeated musical pattern which could be easily recalled. The researcher measured the number of signs and spoken words correctly imitated in a story verse context by children diagnosed with autism. In one condition, signed and spoken words were paired with music (singing). In the other condition, signed and spoken words were paired with rhythmic speech without music. Buday (1995) hypothesized that signs taught with music would result in the correct imitation of more signs and more spoken words than the signed words, which were taught with rhythmic speech.

The results showed that the average number of signs and spoken words correctly imitated during the music condition was significantly higher than the average number of signs imitated during the rhythm condition (Buday 1995). This suggests that music enables a child with autism to focus more intently on on-task behaviors by reducing boredom. During the music condition, the investigator observed fewer stereotyped behaviors such as hand flapping and head movement as well as less incoherent babbling; she also reported that another explanation for the positive results is that music provides a more enjoyable learning situation for many of the children (Buday 1995).

Buday's findings indicate a positive effect of music on sign and speech imitation in children with autism. This effect supports the use of music as an augmentative form of a didactic language intervention (Buday 1995). Her study, however, did not enhance the understanding of how musical patterns influence language acquisition in children with autism. In addition, Buday examined children's imitative ability only. She did not include several critical elements of speech and language development such as pragmatics, semantics, prosody, or phonology in her measurement. In order to understand the positive effect of music on speech and language skills in children with ASD, it is necessary to examine changes in the children's communicative behaviors including use of language after engaging in musical experiences.

If music has such positive effects on enhancing communicative behaviors including speech and language, music stimuli can be used as antecedents for the verbal or nonverbal communicative responses. Braithwaite and Sigafoos (1998) compared the effects of social versus musical antecedents on communication responsiveness in children with developmental disabilities. Children with developmental disabilities and severe communication impairments participated in two antecedent conditions: social interaction or social interaction with a musical antecedent. The social interaction condition consisted of a teacher's initiations of verbal communication, eye contact, and facial expression. The musical antecedent condition consisted of a teacher's singing and acoustic guitar playing with the same social interaction. In each condition, the children were given opportunities to make communication responses such as greeting, naming, and requesting. During the musical antecedent condition, each opportunity was embedded within songs (Braithwaite and Sigafoos 1998).

The results of the study showed moderate increases in communication responsiveness of three children during the musical antecedent condition. In contrast, the other two children had comparable levels of appropriate communicative responding across both conditions. The results suggest that musical antecedents can facilitate communication responsiveness in some children with developmental disabilities. Children were more responsive to the opportunities for greeting and requesting than for naming. Appropriate responding to the naming opportunities was observed for two children who had the highest overall levels of adaptive behaviors among the five children. This finding indicates that the range of communicative intentions expressed by children and their overall functioning levels might be related to social-communicative ability (Braithwaite and Sigafoos 1998).

A number of factors in the music antecedent condition may have influenced the increased communicative behaviors. Motivational and attentional factors in the music had generated greater communicative responsiveness in children with developmental disabilities. Providing opportunities for communicative responses in a musical form (i.e. songs) during the musical antecedent condition can increase the probability of producing previously learned communicative responses (Braithwaite and Sigafoos 1998).

The application of communicative responses learned from musical stimuli in non-musical behaviors of children with ASD need to be examined in order to justify the clinical use of music in ASD treatment. Brownell (2002) investigated the effect of musical social stories on the behaviors of children with autism in four experimental case studies. A social story is a short story that adheres to a specific format and guidelines to objectively describe a person, skill, event, concept, or social situation. A unique social story was created for each child that addressed current target behavior goals, such as eliminating delayed echolalia of movie and television media, following directions, and using a quiet voice. After baseline data collection, the spoken and sung versions of the social stories were alternately presented to the participants using a counterbalanced treatment order (i.e. ABAC/ACAB).

Results from all four case studies indicated that both the spoken version and the sung version were significantly more effective in addressing the target behavior than the control condition. The sung version was significantly more effective than the spoken version in only one case, in which the target behavior was using a quiet voice. Brownell (2002) reported that the frequency of the negative target behaviors, such as excessive talking about TV, displaying difficulty in following directions, and using an intensely loud shouting voice, occurred least often during the presentation of the sung social story. The findings suggest that children with ASD might comprehend a message in a song, and that this comprehension might be enhanced by the perception of patterns in the presented music.

Brownell (2002) suggests that the use of a musical social story is an effective and viable treatment option for modifying behaviors with children with autism. Although the study did not focus on the effect of music on speech and language skills, the findings indicate that both reading and singing a story containing target behavior have a similar beneficial effect on the target behavior. Consequently, children with autism might perceive the musical story and spoken story in a similar manner. Furthermore, they might be able to apply what they learned (or perceived) from either version in their subsequent behaviors.

The positive effects for music in these studies were largely attributed to increased attention, enjoyment, and optimal social context (Brownell 2002; Buday 1995; Hoskins 1988). A close link exists between music and language development in children, and the common perceptual mechanisms for sound might be the primary cause for the link (Hafteck 1997). When speech patterns or elements are paired with a melodic pattern, the speech patterns are easily produced if the melodic pattern is provided as a cue (Buday 1995). Children with autism may prefer certain kinds of music stimuli to other kinds of stimuli because of the repetitiousness and concreteness of the patterns in music (Nelson, Anderson and Gonzales 1984).

The positive effects of music on speech and language in children with ASD have been discussed in recent literature. Some researchers suggest that music improves communicative behaviors in children with ASD, including speech and language. The positive effects of music in the previous studies were largely attributed to increased attention, enjoyment, and optimal social context. However, the inherent musical structures and the neural and perceptual mechanisms in both music and speech might be the reason for the enhanced speech and language.

Part II

Developmental Speech and Language Training through Music for Children with ASD

Clinical Implications and Practice

6

Designing DSLM Protocols

Developmental speech and language training through music (DSLM) utilizes musical elements such as pitch, melody, rhythm, tempo, harmony, form, timbre, dynamics, and instruments in speech and language training for children with language impairments. DSLM is designed to enhance and facilitate speech and language development in children with developmental speech and language delays including children with ASD. In DSLM, other related training materials such as movement, visual, and/or tactile materials are commonly used along with musical materials. Therapeutic music experiences in DSLM can be varied in terms of its therapeutic goal, complexity of the experience, structure of the activity, and utilized materials. However, all therapeutic music exercises in DSLM have to be aligned with developmental scales of normal speech and language in order to be able to engage the child at the appropriate level and help to reach the next developmental level. Knowledge in such areas as first word acquisition, stages of sentence development, semantic development, types of vocabulary acquisition, and length of expected utterances at developmental stages are critical in building creative and emotionally arousing, yet structurally and functionally precise and goal-directed, exercises and experiences (Thaut 2005). This chapter discusses the techniques for designing effective DSLM protocols and skills to compose songs for the protocols.

What kind of songs should we use for DSLM?

Composing songs for DSLM is not an easy task. According to clinical experiences and research findings, the most often produced target words/phrases after music training were located in a few particular songs. The songs for DSLM resulted in more target word/phrase production and were all composed in major keys. The meter of songs and rhythmic figures can be varied upon the number of syllables, prosody, and articulation of the target words/phrases. Target words/phrases should come at the end of each song lyric line. For example, "Hello, hello, *brown bear*. What do you *eat?* I like to eat *apples*. When I eat apples, I am *happy*. Brown bear says, 'I want *more*.' Daddy bear says. 'The apples are *all gone*.'" Each song needs to be composed in a simple structure with a limited number of vocabulary words. If a number of different songs are used in the same DSLM session, each song should be composed in a distinctly different style. For example, the songs varied by key (i.e. C major, F major, D major, E major, D minor, and E minor), tempo, and meter. Songs can be composed in a 4/4 or 2/4 meter, or in 3/4, 6/8, or 12/8 meter. Appendix A has examples of songs for DSLM.

The arrangement of musical elements within the songs needs to be developmentally appropriate for the children. Therefore, all songs must include melodies within a limited pitch range, adjacent intervals, and repetitive melodic contour. Syllabic production (i.e. pronunciation) of the target words/phrases should be emphasized by the rhythmic and harmonic structure as needed to preserve prosody and speech rhythm. Music is composed of many separate yet interconnected components, such as pitch, melody (melodic contour), rhythm, harmony, form,[1] text (lyric), sound quality (timbre), and dynamics[2] (musical prosody). A combination of these musical elements can be perceived as a pattern. The musical patterns in songs for DSLM consist of a variety of elements organized in such a way so as to facilitate the perceptual process and anticipation of information.

Songs for DSLM should be played at a moderate tempo. If the tempo is too fast, it might draw instant attention from the children; however, it might not provide enough time to produce each target word/phrase and to practice the accurate pronunciation. Eventually, the fast tempo of the song

---

1   Musical form uses the terminology of period forms—such terms as phrase, contrasting period, and parallel double period. Commonly these musical forms are described as "binary forms," "ternary forms," "rounded binary forms," etc. In music, a binary form is one that consists of two approximately equivalent sections (therefore, it might consist of a symmetrical pattern in the entire piece of music), although they may be of unequal length. The idea of statement–contrast–return, symbolized as ABA, is an important one in musical form. The ABA, or ternary form, is capable of providing the structure of anything from a short theme to a lengthy movement of a sonata or symphony. The B section of a ternary form can provide a contrast with the A sections by using different melodic material, texture, and tonality, or some combination of these. Binary and ternary forms, especially the latter, provide the structure for many pieces and movements (sections in a whole piece of music) from multimovement/multisection works (Kostka and Payne 2000).

2   Dynamics refers to the expression of musical phrases such as *forte* (*f*—strong) and *piano* (*p*—soft).

will hinder the proper verbal acquisition of the target words/phrases. The song needs to be composed in a parallel period form,[3] in which musical phrases are symmetrically organized. The same melodic contour should be repeated more than twice, and a similar rhythmic figure should be used for all phrases in this song. The pitches in the melodic contour need to be close together, and the same pitches should be used repeatedly. In other words, most of the Gestalt perceptual laws including simplicity, similarity, proximity, good continuation, and completion should be utilized in this song.

The songs composed in a minor key in a slow tempo with a soft dynamic are usually played like a sad lullaby. These songs might not provide the optimal level of stimuli to keep the children's attention for speech and language acquisition. If the form of the song is not symmetrical or parallel, and the melodic contour and pitch movement are repeated infrequently, the temporal patterns in the song might not be predictable. Songs including a chord change from minor to major in the phrase might not utilize the Gestalt laws of perception: simplicity and good continuation. Some of the low functioning children with ASD tend to maintain their attention for the songs that are symmetrical and parallel. The rhythmic patterns of the songs are matched to the syllables of each target word.

Children with ASD might not pay full attention to a song composed in a minor key and played at a slow tempo. They also might not perceive and produce target words/phrases that are embedded in an unpredictable combination of musical patterns in an unsymmetrical structure. Collectively, children with ASD tend to sustain their attention and to respond more favorably to upbeat songs in a major key, than to slow songs in a minor key. Furthermore, children might perceive and produce more linguistic information such as target words/phrases conveyed through the musical patterns of a song in a major key and a fast tempo compared to a song in a minor key and a slow tempo. Children with ASD can perceive and produce target words/phrases that are embedded in simple and repetitive combinations of musical patterns that are symmetrical and parallel in form. The organization of musical patterns via the Gestalt laws might facilitate the perception and subsequent production of target words/phrases conveyed in the musical pattern.

---

3   A parallel period form is applied to a movement or portion of a movement that consists of two main sections.

Clinical implications and techniques for designing DSLM protocols

Children with ASD can improve their speech production after receiving a short-term (i.e. three days) speech and language intervention. Some children with ASD have an intact ability to perceive speech patterns and to produce the speech patterns that contain important linguistic information, including semantics, phonology, pragmatics, and prosody (Lim 2010). This particular finding agrees with previous research indicating that children with ASD clearly have language impairments; however, they may also have an intact ability to perceive and produce speech sounds, and be able to develop some level of functional speech.

Music is an effective method in developmental speech and language training for children with ASD. The children have an intact ability to perceive musical patterns combined with speech patterns, and to produce the speech patterns that contain the same linguistic information in a form of communicational speech language. The demonstrated intact ability of children with ASD to perceive linguistic information has been reported (Heaton *et al.* 1999; Schuler 1995; Tager-Flusberg 1997; Thaut 1999). According to these studies, in spite of dysfunction in auditory-cortical areas in the brain, children with ASD show an intact ability to perceive musical sounds. Organized musical stimuli are perceived by patterns and combined with speech patterns, and this particular pattern perception of music is spared in children with ASD.

Children with speech and language impairment due to ASD can acquire and produce functional vocabulary words by DSLM. This finding can be explained by the common perceptual principle and the mechanism of music and speech in children with ASD. The common perceptual principle is temporal pattern perception through auditory stimuli. In addition, there is a significant integration of the two domains, music and speech, in the language acquisition of children with ASD. In spite of the different characteristics between music and speech stimuli—music is more aesthetic and abstract; speech is more functional and concrete—the perception of musical stimuli might influence speech production by activating the common mechanisms involved in both music and speech. Collectively, children with ASD perceive music and transform the perceived musical patterns into the speech, and then produce functional speech.

The effective strategies for DSLM are as follows:

- listening to songs that contain the functional target words/ phrases

- viewing simplified pictures that correspond to each target word/phrase
- watching a singer's mouth movements while he or she produces each word/phrase
- completing the songs by producing the target words/phrases (i.e. post-testing).

Additional effects from music training might include participants' spontaneous singing (or speaking) while watching the music video. These interventions in the music training resulted in a greater improvement of speech production in children with ASD compared to the speech training. Music training consists of the perception of speech stimuli embedded in musical patterns followed by the production of speech. Speech training consists of the perception of the speech patterns and production of speech.

For music therapy application, listening to songs may be more effective than listening to stories for the acquisition and production of speech components, including semantics, phonology, pragmatics, and prosody of the target words. Utilizing the Gestalt laws of perception (i.e. laws of simplicity, similarity, proximity, common direction, and completion) is the compositional principle for the songs in DSLM.

Children with ASD are able to make an association between auditory stimuli and visual stimuli. During DSLM, target words/phrases are usually presented in a temporal manner with corresponding pictures. As a result, the children can recognize the corresponding pictures, and verbally produce the correctly identified target words/phrases after the training. A music therapist might use visual symbols (i.e. pictures or signs) in speech and language training for children with ASD. Consistent use of visual symbols in DSLM might facilitate literacy in children with ASD including awareness of phonemes and reading comprehension. In order for a child to read and comprehend the symbols, they have to practice the association between auditory and visual stimuli. Auditory and visual association acquired from music or speech and language training could transfer into other functional stimuli such as books, picture schedules, or daily environments.

During the initial stage of DSLM, the music therapist should assess the current language level of the child (i.e. language age, presence of echolalia, and level of functioning), and then select the appropriate category and number of functional vocabulary words and target words/phrases according to the assessment. Next, the music therapist should compose song(s) in a major key and an upbeat tempo with a repeated melodic contour and rhythmic figure. The form of the song should be simple and predictable (i.e. symmetrical), and it is suggested that the target words/phrases be located at the end of lyric lines. The live presentation of musical stimuli is recommended, since the therapist can easily adapt his or her musical performance to the children's response to the music stimuli.

Regardless of the type of training, there should be a consistency and intensity to the speech and language training. It is recommended that training sessions take place on consecutive days, at the same time of the day (more than once a day), and in the same room. Presenting a picture schedule for speech and language training to children with ASD before every training session is recommended. In addition, when the music therapist verbally introduces target words/phrases, presenting the corresponding visual symbols (i.e. picture or sign) is highly recommended. Children with ASD need to practice the association between auditory stimuli (i.e. listening to songs) and visual stimuli (i.e. looking at pictures), in order to enhance further language skills. The music therapist should also encourage the children to sing along while they participate in the speech and language training through music. The music therapist could pause right before each target word/phrase to be sung, and give the children opportunities to complete the lyric lines by singing the target word/phrase. Consistent participation in the developmental speech and language training through music over a long period of time, and repetition of the target word/phrase production, could enhance speech production and language skills in children with ASD.

The clinical foundation for the use of music in speech and language training for children with ASD was discussed. Both music and speech are aural forms of communication. In addition, music and speech share the same acoustical and auditory parameters such as frequency, rhythm, contour, intensity, waveform, timbre, and cadential factor (i.e. principle of good direction and completion). Therefore, carefully designed speech and language training through music might utilize a child's unimpaired ability to perceive music stimuli in order to facilitate speech production.

7

Music Therapy for Speech and Language Development in Children with ASD

Music therapy speech and language training session protocol for children with ASD

This chapter includes the techniques of music therapy speech and language training for children with ASD. The interventions and strategies suggested below are designed for preschoolers (age range three to five) with language deficits due to autism, who are therefore suitable candidates for early autism interventions.

"Goal areas" indicate non-musical behavioral goals and anticipated functional behaviors from the children with ASD. (These goal areas are explained further in the subsection below.) "Musical experiences" include musical stimuli (i.e. antecedent stimuli) provided by music therapists and most relevant musical activities in the particular intervention. Verbal prompts or questions directed by the music therapist can be embedded in singing; therefore they are considered for musical experiences. "Strategies in DSLM" describe specific speech and language training techniques to imply, and how to utilize the example intervention ideas in a clinical music therapy session.

The primary music therapy technique for increasing vocalization and verbalization is to take every opportunity to pair the music therapist's instruction and direction with singing. For example, the music therapist says "This is music time," and then sings *"This is music time, and music is so much fun!"* (The speech should always slightly precede the singing.) Repeat this pairing several times, and if singing is a reinforcer for the child, soon the speech may become reinforcing because it is associated with singing. Therefore, during the early intervention or beginning of the language training, singing the entire instructional stimuli (i.e. verbal stimuli and prompts) can be effective.

Goal areas

Before the interventions are presented, let us elaborate on the "goal area" terms used:

- *Academic skills* are skills involved in school curricula and lesson plans. For example, counting, reading, and writing.

- *Attention / joint attention / selective attention / sustained attention. Attention* is a foundation skill that is necessary for good memory, executive function, communication, and executive control—it is the most important cognitive ability in human functioning. Attention commonly refers to the ability to respond discretely to specific stimuli or activities. *Joint attention* is the process of sharing one's experience of observing an event, by following gaze or pointing gestures. *Selective attention* is the ability to maintain a focus in the face of competing stimuli. *Sustained attention* is the ability to maintain a consistent behavior response during continuous and repetitive activity.

- *Eye contact* is a meeting of eyes between two individuals. It is a form of nonverbal communication.

- *Following direction* is a form of receptive language in speech and language training. It means a response in one's behaviors demonstrating a perceptual understanding of the presented direction in either verbal or nonverbal stimuli and changes in behavior.

- *Group coherence* is an energetic/dynamic phenomenon that occurs in groups when the group accesses its collective identity with a clear sense of the right action to achieve its goals. It is a felt perception, and individuals who have experienced group coherence might recognize it in other contexts and show a certain level of motivation to recreate the experience in other groups.

- *Imagination* is the ability to form mental images, sensations, and concepts in a moment when individuals are not perceived through sight, hearing, or other senses in the presence.

- *Initiation* is the process of starting any change in one's behaviors, including perceptual/cognitive behaviors. It involves the acceptance of both self-perceived behaviors and observed behaviors by others.

- *Intraverbal behavior* is a type of expressive language where a word or phrase evokes another word or phrase, but the two are not identical. For example, the music therapist might have the target words of *bus* and *round* in the song "The Wheels on the Bus Go Round and Round," and then *you* and *me* for the *Barney* "I Love You" song. The child-produced words *bus, round, you,* and *me* are the intraverbal behaviors.

- *Listening to others* is a form of receptive language and involves turn-taking.

- *Matching auditory and visual stimuli* is the process of presenting an identical stimulus in two different sensory modalities. For example, hearing the word "cat" and looking at a picture of a cat.

- *Motor imitation* is the ability to copy and imitate another person's motoric movements, including the shape, feature, duration, interval, and speed of the movements.

- *Movement control* refers to a production of well-coordinated movements. Movement control consists of balance, strength, endurance, flexibility, and overall coordination of movement.

- *Nonverbal communication* is a type of communication not involving words or speech, such as eye contact.

- *Reading skills* are the skills involved in the process of interpreting the written or printed word.

- *Receptive language* is the comprehension of language. It includes the process of listening and understanding what is communicated.

- *Rhythmic entrainment* is the effect of auditory rhythm to synchronize and entrain in the physical movement. Auditory rhythm has an attractor function for movement, which is (1) immediacy and (2) time stability. The physical mechanism for the perception of rhythm is the detection or periodicity patterns in the presented rhythm.

- *Sitting/proper sitting. Proper sitting* is the ability to sustain the original position of *sitting* without any interruption while the stimuli is being presented.

- *Social interaction* is the interplay and/or mutual influence between two or more people and each other's behavior.

- *Story telling* is the telling of a story or a narration of anecdotes, incidents, or fictitious tales.

- *Taking turns* is the back-and-forth interaction in a conversation. Turn-taking is one of the fundamental elements of conversation.

- *Touching others appropriately* indicates an appropriate social manner/behavior demonstrating a close and positive interaction between two individuals.

- *Verbal behavior* refers to applied verbal behavior. It is a methodology that is based upon behavioral principles. The description and explanation of verbal behavior is in Chapter 8.

- *Verbal production* refers to the ability to produce aural sounds through the vocal system—in particular, it refers to speech production.

Intervention 1: Music time orientation song

Goal areas

Verbal behaviors (applied behavior analysis [ABA] verbal behavior), eye contact, rhythmic entrainment, attention, and sitting.

Musical experiences

(A) Singing.

> "*This is music time! This is a fun time! Everybody can sing and play. Everybody is happy.*"

This Is Music Time

Hayoung A. Lim

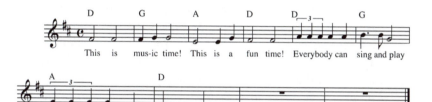

(B) Clapping.

Strategies in DSLM

1. Start every music therapy session with the song. This particular intervention orients the children and notifies them of the beginning of the music therapy session; therefore, it should be placed first in the session schedule. Orienting the music therapy session is an important procedure in any music therapy protocol for children with ASD.

2. Repeat the song at least twice. The consistent repetition of the procedure appears to elicit behaviors indicating increased attention of children with ASD, and improvements in their speech production following the training. Children with ASD also demonstrate these behavior changes and practice effects during the following sessions. The children will show increased attention and familiarity with the song. Familiarity with the stimuli and repetition of stimuli presentation might be a critical factor for producing speech and language in children with ASD.

3. Use live guitar accompaniment. In this intervention, the music therapist should emphasize the various musical components including rhythm, melody, dynamic, form, and instrument in the sounds. Live presentation of such musical components is strongly recommended, since it will increase the children's attention and favorable response.

4. After a couple of repetitions (singing), apply the "intraverbal behavior" techniques. Intraverbal behavior is a type of expressive language where a word or phrase evokes another word or phrase, but the two are not identical. It resembles word association, such as a tendency to say "mouse" when someone says "Mickey." Teaching intraverbal skills begins with selecting a few target words from the songs which the child is familiar with and listens to often. The music therapist sings the songs, pausing just before the target word with the goal of the child filling in the missing word. Once the child masters the last word to several lines from many songs, the music therapist might start backward chaining and leave off the last two words from the sentence. For example, if the child masters "star" when the music therapist sings "Twinkle, twinkle, little _____," the next target would be the phrase "little star." With this chaining technique, the child becomes able to sing the whole song and these intraverbal skills can be transferred to more advanced verbal skills. This particular technique of language acquisition utilizes a common Gestalt law of perception, which involves perceptual completion. The target word in a song placed at the end of each phrase allows the child to anticipate the location and time of the target words to be produced. The structurally and functionally organized singing experience enhances speech production and vocabulary acquisition in children with ASD (Lim 2010).

5. Start intraverbal training with the very last word "Happy" in the song.

   "This is music time! This is a fun time! Everybody can sing and play. Everybody is _____."

6. Try to make a pause after singing "This is _____." If the children comes up with "music time," then approve the answer with the context and make more conversations based on the correct verbal response. For example, "That's right, this is music time. Are you ready to start music time?"

7. Encourage the children to clap (synchronize to music therapist's accompaniment patterns).

8. Use this orientation song in a one-to-one setting.

   "This is music time! This is a fun time! Everybody can sing and play. Michael is happy."

Intervention 2: My name is _____

Goal areas

Verbal production (speech), eye contact, social interaction, touching others appropriately, joint attention, and taking turns.

Musical experiences

(A) Singing.

"My name is _____. I'm happy to meet you! My name is _____. Nice to meet you."

My Name is ____

Hayoung A. Lim

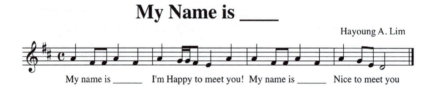

(B) Performing: standing in front of the group and shaking hands with each member of the group.

Strategies in DSLM

1. The music therapist should provide a modeling for this song, and sing for each child's turn.

2. The music therapist uses many gestures and hand motions while singing, for example pointing to herself and shaking hands with the children.

3. During the beginning sessions, the music therapist puts her arm around each child and holds the child's hands to produce both the verbal target word (e.g. name) and nonverbal target gestures (e.g. pointing to himself and shaking hands with each member of the group).

4. After each child completes the song and shaking hands, the music therapist asks the rest of the group "What is his (or her) name?"

5. If there are some children who are starting to learn the alphabet, the music therapist might use a name tag and let each child point to the name tag while singing.

Intervention 3: Singing with the pictures

Goal areas

Intraverbal behavior, matching auditory and visual stimuli, sustained attention, and proper sitting.

Musical experiences

(A) Singing (i.e. Fill-in-the-blank): see Appendix A.

(B) DSLM intraverbal training: as the child develops an intraverbal repertoire, the music therapist can use pictures or photos of the repertoire as visual prompts and facilitate tact training (an ABA verbal behavior) to intraverbal transfer (see Appendix B for the pictures).

Strategies in DSLM

1. Compose songs including the target words/phrases which are located at the end of each lyric line in order to use the DSLM intraverbal technique. For example, "Look at the *pink pig*. He's wearing *shoes*. Oh, where will you *go?*" These songs should be composed in a simple song structure and melodies within a limited pitch range, adjacent intervals, and repetitive melodic contour. The arrangement of musical elements must be developmentally appropriate and syllabic production of the target words/phrases should be emphasized by the rhythm and harmonic structure as needed to preserve prosody and the speech rhythm. Pictures for each target word/phrase should be presented as the music therapist sings the congruent target word/phrase for the tact training.

2. Always start with the music therapist singing the entire text of each song without any prompt and then indicating the children's turn to fill in the blanks. For example, after finishing her singing and presenting the corresponding pictures, the music therapist should say "Now, it's your turn to sing this song with the pictures." The music therapist should start singing the beginning part of each lyric line and make a pause right before the target word/phrase. For example, "*In the morning, the yellow duck likes to* _____."

3. Repetition of the musical and visual presentation can improve the intraverbal skills with picture–vocabulary identification skills.

4. Intraverbal training procedures can be conducted simultaneously with the training of other verbal production including verbal imitation and questioning "What is this?"

5. Live singing is recommended, but recorded accompaniment of the songs can be used, since the music therapist needs to hold and present the corresponding pictures.

6. When the children become familiar with the songs and pictures, the music therapist should ask them to sing the entire song without the antecedent phrases.

7. In order to generalize the effect of DSLM on the speech production, the music therapist might speak the antecedent phrases and ask the children to speak the target words/phrases.

8. This intervention is appropriate for both group and individual sessions.

Intervention 4: Stop and go or "freeze" game

Goal areas

Verbal production (semantics, pragmatics, and prosody), receptive language, following direction, movement control, selective attention, and group coherence.

Musical experiences

(A) Listening to the live or recorded song.

"Shake, shake, shake! Shake, shake, shake, shake. Everybody shake, shake! Ah, ah, ah, ah, ah... Stop. Shake, shake, shake! Shake your shaker [e.g. tambourine, egg shakers, or caterpillar]! Everybody shake, shake! Ah, ah, ah, ah, ah... All done!"

Shake Shake Shake

Hayoung A. Lim

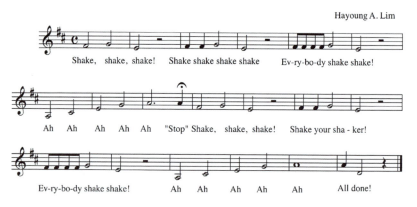

(B) Playing rhythm instruments (e.g. tambourine, egg shakers, or caterpillar).

(C) Watching the visual signs of "Stop" and "Go."

Strategies in DSLM

1. An instrument (i.e. motivational variable), verbal stimuli in the song, and visual signs are required.

2. The song should include multiple opportunities for the children to follow directions (e.g. musical or verbal) indicating when the children should stop and move. The music therapist can provide a live musical direction such as abrupt or anticipated stopping during the song. Verbal direction such as "Stop" in the middle of the song is also recommended.

3. The music therapist should provide either verbal or musical prompts for the children to say "Stop" and "Go." With live music, the music therapist can pause her playing until the children shout "Go." In this way, the children might develop the sense of control along with perceptual anticipation skill. Repetition of this intervention might develop the pattern perception and production skills in children with ASD.

4. When the children become familiar with this intervention, the music therapist assigns a child to be leader of the group. The leader can hold the visual sign and indicate when the rest of the group (including the music therapist) should stop or continue to move.

Intervention 5: What number is this?

Goal areas

Verbal production (semantics, tact, and identification), attention, and academic skills.

Musical experiences

(A) Singing and responding to a song.

First song example: *"What number is this? What number is this?"* *"That's right! This is number one! Thank you very much!"*

What Number is This?

Hayoung A. Lim

What num-ber is this?   What num-ber is this?That's right! This is number one!   Thank you Ve-ry Much!

Second song example: *"This is number three, number three. Can you tell me what is number _____?"*

(B) Verbal prompts in a song.

(C) DSLM-tact (verbal identification) training: presenting the visual stimulus (numbers on card) on the designed rhythm (beats). Tact is the ability to verbally label common items that a child can see, smell, taste, hear, touch, and feel. A tact is associated with the meaning of the vocabulary word; however, this skill is very different from the receptive identification of items or actions. Tacting is a more difficult skill because the child not only must identify the correct word, but also must be able to have the vocal control to independently pronounce the word.

Strategies in DSLM

1. DSLM-tact training begins with presenting a nonverbal stimulus and demanding speech as the response. The antecedent for a tact is some form of nonverbal stimulus (e.g. numbers on cards, or pictures) and the consequence for a tact is positive reinforcement, such as praise (e.g. "That's right!" or "Thank you very much!"), stickers, or the child's favorite activity. Children with autism might learn to produce the target verbal responses fairly quickly because of the positive reinforcement. In tact training, a child is reinforced with praise or some other item or event for being correct in his verbal identification or labeling.

2. Pair the music therapist's instruction and direction with singing. The music therapist starts singing *"This is number time, number time. It is all about numbers, numbers."* The music therapist can direct the children's attention to the visual number cards while singing *"Look at the number and tell me what it is."* If the children cannot produce and identify the target number, the music therapist sings *"This is number five. Everybody, sing with me. Number five, number five, this is number five."* After a couple of repetitions, the music therapist should give another opportunity for the children to verbally identify the target number.

3. If the child wants to hold the number card, the music therapist should give the card and sing *"What number is this?"* or *"This is number __."* When the child correctly responds to the target number, the music therapist asks him to hand the card back to her and sings *"Thank you very much."*

4. When the child becomes familiar with responding to one number at a time, the music therapist might present a couple of different numbers at the same time. (This particular technique might need a desk or a board.) The music therapist asks the child to pick up a target number card among others by singing *"Where is number seven?"* or *"Michael is going to find number seven."* The music therapist should always give praise and/or approval (e.g. positive reinforcement) by singing. For example, *"That's right! This is number seven. Michael found number seven. Good job."*

Intervention 6: Counting song

Goal areas

Verbal production (imitation, intraverbal, and tact), rhythmic entrainment, attention, and academic skills.

Musical experiences

(A) Singing or listening to the recorded song.

First song example: *"One, two, buckle my shoe. Three, four, open the door. Five, six, pick up the sticks. Seven, eight, lay them straight. Nine, ten, do it again!"*

One, Two Buckle my Shoe

Hayoung A. Lim

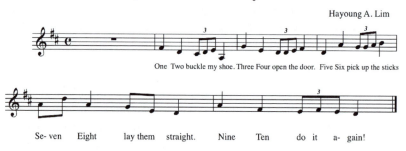

Second song example: *"One, two, button my shirt. Three, four, get in the car. Five, six, sit up straight. Seven, eight, fasten seat belt. Nine, ten, yeah! Let's go."*

Third song example: "*Number one for one ice cream cone. Number two for two blue socks. Number three for three red apples. Number four for four leaf clover. Number five for five little stars. Number six for six singing birds. Number seven for seven jumping mice. Number eight for eight yummy cookies. Number nine for nine sleepy cats. Number ten for ten mighty fingers.*"

Numbers One to Ten

Hayoung A. Lim

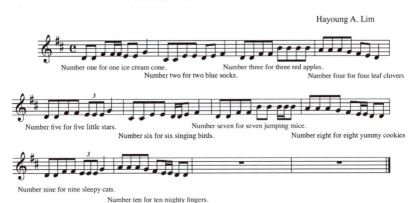

(B) Playing rhythm instruments while counting the numbers.

Sing "*One, two.*" Play instruments (echoing) for two beats: "*One, two.*"

Sing "*Three, four, five.*" Play instruments for three beats: "*Three, four, five.*"

Sing "*Six, seven, eight, nine.*" Play instruments for four beats: "*Six, seven, eight, nine.*"

Sing "*And ten.*" Play instruments for multiple beats: "*Te--------------n.*"

Strategies in DSLM

1. Utilize the verbal stimuli in the song and nonverbal stimuli (e.g. number on flash card). If the music therapist uses a recorded song, she can present the cards and repeat the verbal prompts. If this is the very first time of use, the music therapist might just play the song and present the materials without giving the children any opportunity to respond. Then, the music therapist sings the song live, considers the appropriate pace (e.g. tempo) for the children, and provides many verbal prompts. When the children start to count and/or correctly respond to some of the stimuli, the music therapist should play the recorded song again.

2. Use musical instruments such as rhythm sticks or a drum for counting. Pairing the verbal counting and movement might give the children the incident feedback for correct counting and allow them to develop a rhythm pattern production skill that is critical for their speech and language development.

3. The children should be encouraged to sing the entire song by imitation or memory. Although they seem to sing by imitating the lyrics without analyzing the meaning of them (i.e. Gestalt style of language), their spontaneous verbal production in singing should be encouraged. The children might randomly recite the counting song after the intervention or out of the music therapy session. The music therapist or parents should reinforce this particular behavior by singing and counting with the children and/or showing the number cards. These types of reinforcement or approval will develop the appropriate perceptual association between the simple imitative singing and counting numbers. Singing the counting song becomes a positive reinforcement for the children to produce the verbal counting of numbers.

4. When the children show the ability to count all the numbers with one particular song, the music therapist should attempt to change some lyrics or the song or introduce a new counting song. The change of the lyrics in a counting song will increase the generalization of the verbal production and learning numbers for children with ASD. The music therapist can simply change a couple of words in the song. For example, "*One, two, button my shirt. Three, four, get in the car. Five, six, sit up straight. Seven, eight, fasten seat belt. Nine, ten, yeah! Let's go.*"

Intervention 7: Group ensemble

Goal areas

Verbal production (requesting or mand operant), listening to others, receptive language, selective attention, and social interaction.

Musical experiences

(A) Listening and responding to a song.

First song example: *"Everybody play, play, play, play your instrument. Everybody play, play, play, play your instrument." "Let me hear Vicky [each child's name], Vicky, Vicky playing her instrument." "Vicky can play, play, play, play the rhythm sticks!"*

Everybody Play your Instrument!

Hayoung A. Lim

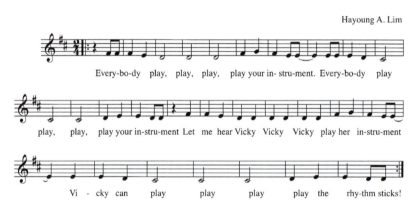

Second song example: *"We are great young musicians. We are great young musicians. We are great young musicians. Everybody plays music together." "Michael [each child's name] plays the tambourine [instrument the child is holding]. Michael plays the tambourine. Michael plays the tambourine. Oh, he sounds so good!"*

We are Great Young Musicians

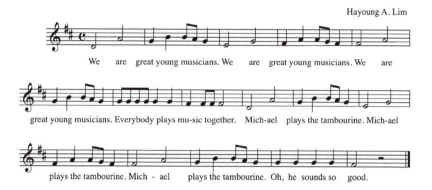

Hayoung A. Lim

We   are   great young musicians. We   are   great young musicians. We   are

great young musicians. Everybody plays mu-sic together.   Mich-ael   plays the tambourine. Mich-ael

plays the tambourine. Mich - ael   plays the tambourine. Oh, he sounds so   good.

(B) Verbal prompts for requesting (i.e. mand).

"What do you want to play?" or *"Which instrument do you want to play?"*; and for identifying (i.e. tact): *"What does Vicky play?"*

(C) Playing various instruments in an ensemble.

Strategies in DSLM

1. A child's ability to verbally request, which is commonly referred to as "mand operant," is important in his or her speech and language development. This ability is usually controlled by what children want or by a motivational variable. Thus, the music therapist should determine and design the intervention so the children can present their needs and desires. A successful intervention to teach requesting skills should indicate the children's ability to request, and can predict a training effect of motivational reinforcers such as their favorite musical instruments. Normally developing children acquire this verbal skill quite quickly without much instruction; however, children with autism have deficits in learning how to use words to ask for what they want.

2. Many young children with autism do not usually request objects or items that they obviously want, which indicates that they do not use language to control their environment for their own benefit. Musical instruments could be used as an effective form of reinforcement for the children, and the ability to verbally request the reinforcers allows them control over their environment. This control that children gain over their social environment such as a group ensemble should increase the value of language training in general, increase responsiveness to language, and the ability to initiate first words, and begin to establish the speaker and listener roles that are essential to further verbal development. Requesting a musical instrument should be produced spontaneously, and the generalization may occur quickly because of the unique effects of the motivational reinforcement (e.g. having the instrument after verbally requesting it).

3. The initial training should begin with use of all the antecedent variables including motivational instruments and verbal prompts (e.g. questions by the music therapist). In order to conduct a group ensemble for speech and language training, the music therapist should present a couple of different musical instruments to the children. However, the initial trial for this intervention will consist of the music therapist holding up an instrument (e.g. drum) and saying or singing to each child, "What do you want to play?" (i.e. verbal stimulus to respond), and "Say drum" (i.e. echoic stimulus). If the child produces an approximation of the word "drum" immediately, the music therapist delivers praise or physical contact and a drum (i.e. specific reinforcement as a consequence). No response or an incorrect response should be followed by a re-presentation of the previous trial. If the child continues to fail to respond, the instructor might try a different instrument when the child's motivation is stronger, or consider the use of sign language or picture communication in the early stage of training.

4. The procedure for actual training begins as the echoic stimulus or imitative prompts (e.g. "Say drum") are phased out. After the successful trials without the echoic prompt, the music therapist should ask "What do you want to play?" If the child says "drum," the drum will be immediately delivered to the child. The last step is to phase out the verbal question to the response. The music therapist simply introduces: "Now, it is time to play the instruments." When the child wants to play the drum, he or she will say "drum" and the instrument will be immediately delivered.

5. While conducting the group ensemble, the music therapist should give each individual child and the group a very clear direction with active verbal prompts such as "It is Jenny's turn. Only Jenny plays rhythm sticks. If you are not Jenny, don't play" and "Wait for your turn. I will let you know when everybody can play." After one child's playing, the music therapist should ask the group "Which instrument did Jenny play?" If the children cannot respond correctly (e.g. rhythm sticks), the music therapist sings *"Let's hear Jenny playing rhythm sticks, rhythm sticks."* The children might be eager to play instruments on their turn, and they understand that giving the correct answer will shorten the waiting time. In addition, the music therapist should always give praise after each child's turn to play in the ensemble and any of the children's verbal responses.

6. Alternating individual children's turns and everybody's chance of playing in a trial is an effective technique to teach selective attention and turn-taking skills in daily communication.

7. The music therapist should facilitate this particular ensemble intervention with live singing and accompaniment in order to provide appropriate verbal prompts and directions.

8. For DSLM, various musical experiences such as listening to a favorite song, playing favorite instruments, alternating dynamics in musical playing, and moving or dancing to music are used for the

motivational variables in verbal requesting skill (i.e. mand) training. Target words/phrases might include various vocabularies such as "song," "sing," "play," "fast," "slow," "stop," "go," "hand," "dance," "all done," "finished," "my turn," and "music," the names of instruments, the titles of songs, and the names of music activities. If the child verbally requests any of the reinforcers, the music therapist must provide the item or facilitate the particular musical experiences. Eventually, the music therapist asks or sings "What do you want to play today?" or "How do you want to sing?" and the child might answer with "drum" or "fast and loud."

Intervention 8: Alphabet letter song

Goal areas

Verbal production (intraverbal and tact), attention, reading skills, and academic skills.

Musical experiences

(A) Singing.

"A for the Apple, B for the Baby, C for the Cat…"

(B) Verbal prompts for tact.

"What letter is this?" with letter on flash card.

Alphabet

Hayoung A. Lim

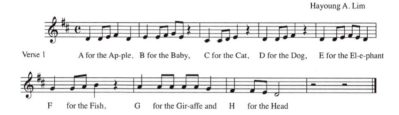

Verse 1   A for the Ap-ple, B for the Baby,   C for the Cat,   D for the Dog,   E for the El-e-phant

F   for the Fish,   G   for the Gir-affe and   H   for the Head

Verse 2: *"I for the Igloo, J for the Jar, K for the Key, L for the Leaf, M for the Mask, N for the Nail, O for the Owl, and P for the Pig."*

Verse 3: *"Q for the Queen, R for the Rake, S for the Snail, T for the Table, U for the Umbrella, V for the Violin, W for the Whale, and X for the Xylophone."*

After verse 3: *"Y is for Yellow, and Z is for Zipper."*

(C) Drawing with singing.

"What does Mister A look like? Let's draw Mister A. Up and down and cross. Mister A looks like letter A." "What does Mister B look like? Let's draw Mister B. Down line and two half circles. Mister B looks like letter B."

Mister A

Hayoung A Lim

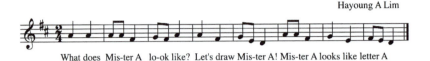

What does Mis-ter A lo-ok like? Let's draw Mis-ter A! Mis-ter A looks like letter A

Strategies in DSLM

1. Functional vocabulary words such as alphabet letters can be produced with a combination of musical elements. Functional and concrete speech (i.e. words) might be integrated into music, and the perceived musical patterns may facilitate speech production. The particular combination of musical elements is usually organized in a repetitive and predictable manner that is perceived as a pattern. Repetition of the predictable temporal patterns in a simple song may increase attention and elicit anticipation for the subsequent musical patterns within the structure. Furthermore, anticipation for the musical pattern may enhance the children's further cognitive processes such as association or recall of the words embedded in a song.

2. The music therapist should compose a few distinctive melodies for this intervention. Each phrase or melody should be composed with a melodic contour combined with a simple rhythmic configuration, so the phrase is perceived as a musical pattern (i.e. unit). The melodic contour was organized in its simplest form; this particular melodic contour with a simple rhythmic configuration should be repeated in each song. The organization of the repeated melody lines with similar rhythmic patterns in the letter song might develop familiarity in the children. In addition, the pitches of the melody are relatively close together. The step-wise pitch movement might be perceived as a pattern. For example, adjacent pitches associated with the target alphabet letter and word (A for the Apple: C-C-D-E-C; B for the Baby: D-D-E-F) help the grouping of the letters and words. The pitches and rhythmic figures also need to be matched to the syllables of each target word. As a result, the combination

of musical elements and target words will be perceived as a whole unit. The described organization of musical patterns, therefore, enhances the children's anticipation and prediction, and supports their perceptual process of alphabet letters and words presented with the musical patterns.

3. The timely presentation of the visual letters and words (items) on a flash card is strongly suggested. It is also suggested that the music therapist hand each flash card out to the child, when she sings the corresponding phrase, so the child can develop a more active perceptual association between the visual letter and the sounds.

4. For intraverbal training, the music therapist can make a pause right before the vocabulary word. For example, the music therapist sings "*A for the _____*" and waits for the child to fill in the blank by saying or singing "Apple." In addition, the music therapist can hold the flash card and ask the child to name the alphabet letter. If the child says "B," the music therapist fills in the blank by singing "*for the Baby.*" This particular technique will develop conversational and turn-taking skills in a real dialogue in children with ASD. Many children with autism show difficulty in answering questions and participating in meaningful conversations, despite having the ability to speak hundreds of vocabulary words. Conversational skills consist of intraverbal behaviors which are important for social interaction, as well as for the acquisition of academic skills.

5. When the music therapist facilitates the drawing activity in this DSLM intervention, it is recommended to compose and memorize all of the lyrics prior to the session. The main music therapy technique in this particular intervention is to describe the shape or feature of each alphabet letter in a melody. The music therapist might need to use lots of onomatopoeias or random speech sounds to describe the shape of the letter. For example, "*What does Mister S look like? Let's draw Mister S. Siss, siss, like a snake moves. Mister S looks like letter S.*"

6. The music therapist should try to pair her instructions and directions with singing. In addition, it is suggested that the children sing the directions as they draw the letter. After the children complete the

drawing of each letter, the music therapist needs to sing "*What letter is this? What letter is this? Can you tell me what letter this is?*" to give them the opportunities to verbally identify the letter.

7.   The music therapist can also use the children's own drawings for further letter identification training. Children might have better perceptual association and congruity toward the letters they have produced on the paper. The music therapist can modify and sing the song for this particular technique: "*What does Mister A look like? Let's look at Mister A. Up and down and cross. Mister A looks like letter A.*" "*What does Mister B look like? Let's look at Mister B. Down line and two half circles. Mister B looks like letter B.*" The children will watch their own drawing and identify the corresponding letter.

Intervention 9: Shake your beanbag!

Goal areas

Verbal production (tact and mand), motor imitation, receptive language, and social interaction.

Musical experiences

(A) Singing and responding to the song.

First song example: *"Hold your beanbag on your head. Hold your beanbag on your shoulder. Now hold your beanbag and shake it loud!"* *"Hold your beanbag on your knee. Hold your beanbag on your tummy. Now hold your beanbag and throw it to the sky."*

Hold Your Beanbag

Hayoung A. Lim

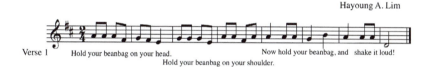

Verse 1   Hold your beanbag on your head.   Now hold your beanbag, and   shake it loud!
                 Hold your beanbag on your shoulder.

Second song example: *"I'm gonna shake my beanbag [or shaker] on my knee. I'm gonna shake my beanbag on my elbow. I'm gonna shake my beanbag on my head and be happy all day long!"*

Verse 2: *"Hold your beanbag on your knee. Hold your beanbag on your tummy. Now hold your beanbag and throw it to the sky."*

Shake My Beanbag

Hayoung A. Lim

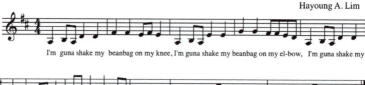

I'm guna shake my beanbag on my knee, I'm guna shake my beanbag on my el-bow, I'm guna shake my

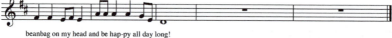

beanbag on my head and be hap-py all day long!

(B) Verbal prompt for mand.

"What color of beanbag do you want?"; or tact: *"What color is this?"*

(C) Verbal prompt for mand.

"Where should we shake our beanbags?"; or tact-intraverbal: *"I'm gonna shake my beanbag on my _____"* (and pointing to a particular body part).

Strategies in DSLM

1. For the first trial, the music therapist should repeat the singing and demonstrate all of the corresponding movements. In this trial, the use of three or four body parts is suggested. If the children copy the music therapist's movements including holding beanbags, shaking beanbags, throwing beanbags, and catching beanbags, the music therapist may start teaching one verb (e.g. hold, shake, throw, and catch) at one time by singing with movement demonstration. For example, the music therapist can sing *"Hold your beanbag, hold your beanbag. Now, it is time to hold your beanbag."* Then, she can continue to sing *"Shake your beanbag, shake your beanbag. Now, it is time to shake your beanbag."*

2. This particular intervention can be started with a song for body part identification such as *"Head and shoulder, knee and toe, knee and toe."* Orienting the children with different body parts might help them to apply the identification skill in the beanbag activity.

3. The music therapist can provide different kinds of verbal prompts for this intervention including *"What color beanbag do you want?"* or *"Where should we shake our beanbags?"* It is important to give children many opportunities to verbally respond while participating in this intervention.

4. When the children have completed the intervention (e.g. follow all of the directions in singing, and perform all of the movements), the music therapist can use a picture (of a child) for them to identify different body parts by placing their beanbags on the picture. The music therapist can sing *"Put your beanbag on David's [name of a boy in the picture] head. Put your beanbag on David's arm,"* and then sing *"Take your beanbag from David's head. Take your beanbag from David's arm."* This particular technique will develop the children's receptive language as well as joint attention. If the group members are familiar to each other and not avoiding touching each other, the music therapist may use each child in the group to implement this technique. It will be also a valuable experience for each individual child with ASD to directly interact and make contact with someone else.

5. Another technique to implement with this intervention is teaching spatial concepts and preposition in language. If the child or children show fair receptive language skills for the intervention and the ability to verbally identify and produce the target words (e.g. body parts and verbs for movements), the music therapist may try to teach the use of preposition in receptive and expressive language. Song examples include *"Hold your beanbag on your head. Now place your beanbag on the white desk,"* *"Hold your beanbag under your leg. Now place your beanbag under the blue chair,"* *"Shake your beanbag with your hands. Now put your beanbag in the yellow box,"* or *"Take your beanbag out of the box. Now throw your beanbag and catch it."* Extra verbal prompts which emphasize the preposition and location in the direction are needed. This technique may be more effective for an individual session, since it is receptive language training and lots of extra verbal prompts are necessary.

6. In order to facilitate the expressive language (i.e. speech) training for the use of preposition and indication of location, the music therapist might use the following technique. The music therapist places a couple of beanbags (with different colors) in different

locations such as "under the chair," "on top of the shelf," "in the box," or "in the drawer." The child should see where the music therapist places those beanbags in order to verbally respond. After placing the beanbags, the music therapist will sing *"Where is the yellow beanbag? Where is the yellow beanbag? Michael can tell you where it is."* The correct response will be that the child says "under the chair." If the child goes to the chair and picks up the yellow beanbag, the music therapist will sing *"The yellow bag was under the chair and Michael found it,"* and give another opportunity for him to say "under the chair."

Intervention 10: Let's play drum

Goal areas

Verbal production (mand and verbal imitation), motor imitation, initiation, nonverbal communication, and social interaction.

Musical experiences

(A) Producing rhythmic patterns in playing drums.

(B) Alternating dynamics in playing drums.

(C) Singing.

"*If Audrey plays _____, Michael plays _____.*"

"*Fast and loud,*" or "*Slow and soft.*"

(D) Verbal prompt for mand: "*How do you want to play?*"

Strategies in DSLM

1. The music therapist may start this intervention by giving the child an opportunity to play the drum without much direction. It is suggested that the music therapist let the child explore his or her musical creativity and pattern production skills. After exploring the random drum playing, the music therapist starts singing "*Fast and loud, fast and loud. We play the drum fast and loud*" and plays her drum very fast and loud. If the child joins in playing the drum fast and loud, the music therapist reinforces the playing with continuous singing and playing. The music therapist should stop singing and playing the drum fast and loud after 30 seconds and make a strong eye contact with the child while slowly singing "*Slow and soft*" and playing the drum slow and soft. If the child joins in playing the drum slow and soft, the music therapist reinforces his playing with continuous singing and playing. The music therapist should stop singing and playing the drum slowly and softly after 30 seconds, and ask the child "Now, how would you like to play the drum, fast and loud or slow and soft?" Most of the children will answer "fast

and loud." The music therapist should verbally approve the child's answer and immediately sing and play the drum fast and loud.

2. This intervention utilizes imitation skills in children with ASD and develops verbal imitation skill commonly called "echoic" skill. The echoic operant involves repeating what someone else says, similar to an echo. A child's ability to repeat sounds and words (i.e. echoic behavior) plays a very important role in language acquisition and speech development. Information regarding the quality and strength of the echoic repertoire from vocal imitation can reveal potential problems in producing response topographies that are essential for other verbal interactions. If the child cannot echo specific sounds, the probability of those responses occurring in other functional units of verbal behavior is quite low. If a nonverbal child cannot repeat any sounds or words, the child may be a candidate for the use of sign language or augmentative communication devices.

3. The ultimate goal of this training is to increase the child's spontaneous use of speech, and to bring specific vocalization or verbalization under imitative control. The first procedure in the training involves the use of direct reinforcement for any vocalization or verbalization of the child, so that the frequency of the verbal production and reinforcement might be increased. The instruction in echoic training should begin with a sound that the child has produced frequently in the past. The procedure consists of presenting the child with the verbal prompt "say…" or the musical prompt "sing…" and reinforcing a correct response, since the child needs to produce the specific sound on command. If the child cannot imitate the vocal sounds, the music therapist should use the drum. The music therapist should play a very simple rhythm pattern on a drum and then give a drum stick to the child. Physical prompts such as holding the drum stick with the child is recommended if the child cannot play the drum spontaneously. The correct response is that the child copies the exact rhythm pattern on the drum.

4. An effective technique in echoic training is utilizing turn- taking activities. The music therapist sings "*If Audrey [name of the therapist] says hello, Michael [name of the child] says hello*" and then repeats the line with "*If Audrey says hello, Michael says* _____." If the child says "hello" within the singing by himself, the music therapist says

"hello." The child might imitate the entire phrase or imitate only "hello." Appropriate social reinforcements such as praise, hi-five, or stickers are often effective for further verbal imitation. In drum playing the same turn-taking technique is suggested. The music therapist should sing and play "*If Audrey plays pom, pom [with the actual drum beats], Michael plays pom, pom,*" and "*If Audrey plays pom, pom, pom, Michael plays pom, pom, pom.*" After teaching the rule (turn-taking), the music therapist should start singing and playing "*If Audrey plays _____, Michael plays _____.*" Having two separate drums for the music therapist and the child is suggested as the intervention becomes familiar to the child.

5. The echoic training with music should target the child's initiation in interaction. If the child is familiar with the echoic training with turn-taking, the music therapist gives the child opportunities to initiate. For example, the music therapist starts singing "*If Michael says Tika Tika, Audrey says Tika Tika*" while indicating each turn (i.e. pointing to the child and then pointing to the music therapist), and then sings "*If Michael says _____*" and waits a few seconds. When the child comes up with his or her sounds including "*Tika Tika,*" the music therapist immediately sings "*Audrey says _____,*" repeating the sounds the child produced. This technique should be implemented with the drum intervention. Being familiar with the various rhythmic patterns is necessary for the child to participate in this intervention. Commonly, children with ASD show a difficulty initiating and producing new rhythmic patterns. While initiating rhythms they tend to produce a set beat pattern (mostly the first pattern they produced) and not change the pattern for the following trials. In this case, the music therapist should let the child know that the rhythm pattern is the same, and refuse to imitate the child's pattern. If the child shows a small change in his or her playing, the music therapist should immediately copy the pattern with exaggerating the change. This particular training can be further developed into other types of speech and language training, making a dialogue, call and response, and musical ensemble, so that the child becomes engaged in a more spontaneous initiation for communication and social interaction.

Intervention 11: Dance like an animal

Goal areas

Verbal production (identification and intraverbal), imagination, motor imitation, and initiation.

Musical experiences

(A) Singing.

"We're gonna dance like an animal, dance like an animal. Dance like an elephant, dance like an elephant, everyone dance like an elephant!"

Dance Like an Animal

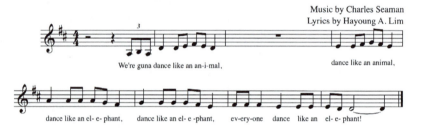

Music by Charles Seaman
Lyrics by Hayoung A. Lim

We're guna dance like an an-i-mal,   dance like an animal,

dance like an el- e- phant,   dance like an el- e -phant,   ev-ery-one   dance   like an   el- e- phant!

(B) Listening and creating different sounds (musical sounds describing animals' movements).

(C) Movement to music.

Strategies in DSLM

1. The music therapist should introduce this intervention by singing *"We're gonna dance like an animal, dance like an animal,"* and ask the children "What animal do you want to pick?" At the beginning of the session, it is recommended to give two options of a familiar animal for the children to choose with the pictures of animals. For example, the music therapist can ask "Do you want to dance like an elephant

or a lion?" It is strongly suggested to give a clear direction to choose with specific options for children with ASD during most of the interventions. This technique will empower the children to control their following learning experiences and environment. In addition, giving an option to choose might provide the children with greater opportunities to communicate and/or initiate communication in the training spontaneously to interact with others. For children with autism to be judged as socially competent during communicative interactions, spontaneous initiations are necessary. In this intervention, the children will initiate the teaching situation by gesturing or indicating an interest in a desired animal or movement. The children's response of "elephant" will be rewarded with access to the desired experience; that music therapist sings *"Dance like an elephant, dance like an elephant, everybody dance like an elephant."*

2. The piano or keyboard is the most efficient instrument to facilitate this intervention. The music therapist should compose brief melodies and/or sound effects that describe different kinds of movements. If the music therapist and the children decide a movement for the animal dance, the music therapist should demonstrate the movement with a verbal prompt: "We are going to move like this." And then the music therapist provides the musical sounds on the keyboard with the following verbal prompt: "This movement sounds like this. Everybody listen to the sounds and move to the sounds."

3. When the children can imitate and produce the movement, the music therapist should give a verbal question such as "How do you want to move?" It is also suggested to provide an option (e.g. "up," "down" or "fast," "slow") for the children to choose and to implement their responses into the intervention. The music therapist can sing *"We go up, up, up and down, down, down"* to facilitate their new movements.

4. In order to elicit more verbal production during this intervention, the music therapist needs to ask a few questions such as "How did we move?" or "What animal did we dance like?" The music therapist should also encourage the children to sing along while they move.

Intervention 12: Singing book

Goal areas

Verbal production (tact and intraverbal), story telling, sustained attention, reading skills, and academic skills.

Musical experiences

(A) Singing stories in a book.

First song example: *"Ten little monkeys jumping on the bed. One fell off and bumped his head. Mama called the doctor and doctor said, No more monkeys jumping on the bed!"*

Ten Little Monkeys

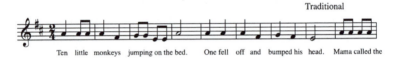

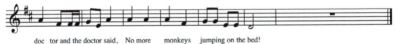

Second song example: *"Brown bear, brown bear, what do you see? I see a red bird looking at me. Red bird, red bird, what do you see? I see a yellow duck looking at me. Yellow duck, yellow duck, what do you see? I see a white dog looking at me."*

Brown Bear

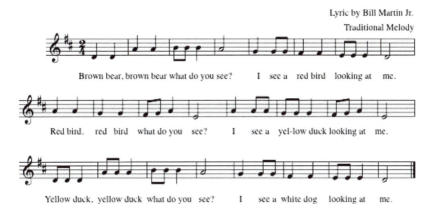

(B) Describing pictures in singing.

"Brown bear is looking at you." "A yellow giraffe is driving Daddy's red car."

(C) Improvisational singing.

(D) Vocal expression.

"What sound does a chicken make? Cluck, cluck, cluck."

Strategies in DSLM

1. The music therapist should compose melodies for each line in a book. Children with ASD perceive and produce the linguistic information from music as they do from speech. Therefore, the music therapist should utilize the Gestalt principles of perceptual organization, such as the principles of pattern perception and recognition, in composing a sing with story lines in the book. The verbal information (story) needs to be embedded properly in a song. Each phrase of the story needs to be composed with a melodic contour combined with a simple rhythmic configuration, so the phrase will be perceived as a musical pattern (i.e. unit). The melodic

line needs to be organized in its simplest form and the pitches of the melodies need to be close together. The pitches and rhythmic figures also need to be matched to the syllables of each word in the story. The combination of musical elements and words in the story line should be perceived as a whole unit.

2. The word at the end of each phrase or story line needs to be emphasized with a proper cadence and a relatively longer note duration. The predictable harmonic progression of each cadence and/or subtle changes in timing (i.e. rubato) on the last note of each phrase will increase the perception of the story line. This compositional technique allows the children to anticipate the location and time of the words to be produced. The described organization of musical patterns will enhance the children's musical anticipation and prediction, and support their perceptual process of the story presented with the musical patterns.

3. When the music therapist establishes the song for a book and the children become familiar with this intervention, the music therapist should apply intraverbal communication, a form of fill-in-the-blank. Intraverbal communication is a type of expressive language in which a word or phrase evokes another word or phrase by cueing or prompting, but the cue is not identical to the response (target word/ phrase). This singing book intervention might provide the optimal training structure to implement the intraverbal communication technique. The music therapist should start presenting the book and singing "*Brown bear, brown bear, what do you* _____?" and then make a pause right before the word at the end of the line. If the children sing or speak "see," the music therapist should continue presenting the book and singing "*I see a red bird looking at* _____."

4. Excessive redundancy of using the same book and song can cause non-beneficial training effects. Children with ASD might produce framed answers and throw a tantrum if the book or song is presented in a missed order. In order to prevent this problem, the music therapist should use various books for this intervention. There are so many good children's books on the market, the music therapist should be able to select books that contain many functional

vocabulary words and stories with regular, well-organized speech patterns. It is suggested to make a picture schedule of the "singing book" (not making the title of the schedule with the title of the book), and alternate different books for this particular schedule.

5. Reading and listening to an entire book requires extensive attention from the children. In addition, producing the target words/ phrases with the correct pragmatic (timing and location of the word production) and semantic skills might be challenging for the children. Therefore, the music therapist should praise any of their verbal productions and provide positive reinforcements (e.g. edibles, favorite musical activity, or finishing the session).

8

DSLM in an Applied Behavior Analysis Verbal Behavior Approach for Children with ASD

This chapter explores the use of DSLM in treating children with ASD within applied behavior analysis (ABA) verbal behavior (VB) approaches, and augments the understanding of empirical mechanisms of language training techniques with music. The chapter discusses the theoretical orientation and major principles of ABA VB approaches that resulted from Skinner's (1957) analysis of verbal behavior for language training. Music's suitability for incorporation with ABA VB approaches is demonstrated in terms of its functions as an automatic reinforcement. Antecedent variables of verbal behaviors including a motivational variable (i.e. establish operation), verbal stimuli, verbal prompts, and nonverbal stimuli are presented. This chapter provides the theoretical and clinical implications of the use of music in ABA VB training by presenting various strategies for using music in language assessment and training. These clinical implications include an example of a music therapy language training session protocol with various music activities that can enhance verbal and nonverbal communicative behaviors in young children with ASD. The ABA VB approach in DSLM is outlined in Table 8.1.

Table 8.1 ABA VB in DSLM

DSLM interventions	Protocol	Antecedent variable	Verbal behaviors	Nonverbal behavior	Session format
Music time orientation song	Singing "*This is music time! This is a fun time! Everybody can sing and play. Everybody is happy.*" Clapping	Musical stimuli in the song and accompaniment (i.e. motivational stimuli) Verbal stimuli and prompts in the song	Mand Echoic Intraverbal	Eye contact Rhythmic entrainment Attention Sitting	Group or individual
My name is ____	Singing "*My name is ____. I'm happy to meet you! My name is ____. Nice to meet you.*" Performing	Musical stimuli (i.e. automatic reinforcement) Verbal stimuli and prompts in the song	Echoic Intraverbal	Eye contact Social interaction Touching others appropriately Joint attention Taking turns	Group

Activity	Description	Stimuli	Verbal operants	Skills	Group or individual
Singing with the pictures	Singing (i.e. Fill-in-the-blank) DSLM intraverbal training	Verbal stimuli in songs Visual stimuli (i.e. prompts)	Intraverbal Tact	Matching auditory and visual stimuli Sustained attention Proper sitting	Group or individual
Stop and go or "freeze" game	Listening to the live or recorded song Playing rhythm instruments Watching the visual signs of "Stop" and "Go"	Instrument (i.e. motivational variable) Verbal stimuli in the song Nonverbal stimuli (i.e. visual signs)	Mand Echoic	Movement control Receptive language Following direction Selective attention Group coherence	Group or individual
What number is this?	Singing and responding to a song *"What number is this?"* Verbal prompts in a song DSLM-tact (verbal identification) training	Verbal stimuli or prompts in a song Nonverbal stimuli (i.e. number on flash card)	Echoic Tact	Attention Academic skills	Individual

DSLM interventions	Protocol	Antecedent variable	Verbal behaviors	Nonverbal behavior	Session format
Counting song	Singing or listening to the recorded song *"One, two, buckle my shoe. Three, four, open the door."* Playing rhythm instruments while counting the numbers	Verbal stimuli in the song Nonverbal stimuli (i.e. number on flash card)	Echoic Tact Intraverbal	Rhythmic entrainment Attention Academic skills	Group or individual
Group ensemble	Listening and responding to a song *"Everybody play, play, play, play your instrument."* *"Let me hear Vicky, Vicky, Vicky play the rhythm sticks."*	Verbal stimuli in the song Verbal prompt for mand: *"What do you want to play?"*; or for tact: *"What does Vicky play?"* Instruments (i.e. nonverbal stimuli and EO)	Mand Tact Echoic	Listening to others Receptive language Selective attention Social interaction	Group
Alphabet letter song	Singing *"A for the Apple, B for the Baby, C for the Cat . . ."*	Musical stimuli in the song (i.e. EO) Verbal prompt for tact: *"What letter is this?"* Nonverbal stimuli (i.e. letter on flash card)	Tact Intraverbal	Attention Reading skills Academic skills	Group or individual

Shake your beanbag!	Singing and responding to the song *"Hold your beanbag on your head."*	Musical stimuli (i.e. EO) Verbal stimuli in the song Instruments (i.e. motivational variables and nonverbal stimuli) Verbal prompt for mand: *"What color do you want?"*; or tact: *"What color is this?"*	Mand Tact	Motor imitation Receptive language Social interaction	Group or individual
Let's play drum **Let's dance**	Alternating dynamics in playing drums Singing *"Fast and loud"* or *"Slow and soft."* *"We go up, up, up and down, down, down."*	Musical stimuli (i.e. EO) Instrument (i.e. motivational variable) Verbal prompts for mand: *"How do you want to play?"* or *"How do you want to move?"*	Mand Echoic	Motor imitation Initiation Nonverbal communication Social interaction	Group or individual
Singing book	Singing stories in a book *"Ten little monkeys jumping on the bed."* *"Brown bear, brown bear, what do you see?"*	Verbal stimuli in singing Nonverbal stimuli (i.e. books)	Tact Intraverbal Story telling	Sustained attention Reading skills Academic skills	Group or individual

Behavior and language training in ASD

Communication difficulties in autism typically are compounded by significant impairments in social interaction and appropriate behaviors. Children may use aberrant behaviors for communication purposes when they lack the appropriate skills to communicate (Chung et al. 1995; Sigafoos 2000). To address both the communication and behavioral needs of children with ASD, researchers and practitioners have investigated numerous interventions and treatment approaches. Intervention or treatment approaches for enhancing social communication abilities for children with ASD vary greatly, and they range in a continuum from traditional discrete trials to more contemporary behavioral approaches that utilize naturalistic language teaching techniques, as well as developmental approaches.

Discrete trial teaching methods for children with ASD

The earliest approaches to teaching speech and language to children with autism were discrete trial teaching (DTT) methods, which utilized didactic methods to teach verbal behavior. Lovaas (1977) is generally credited with introducing the use of DTT techniques for the treatment of speech in autism during the 1970s and 1980s and providing the most detailed account of the procedures for language training using traditional behavioral approaches. Participation in intensive DTT interventions at a very early age resulted in some children with autism making significant improvements (Green, Brennan and Fein 2002). It has been suggested that DTT approaches can be an effective means of initially developing attention to and understanding of language, as well as initiating speech production in pre-verbal children with ASD (Paul and Sutherland 2005). However, the lack of spontaneity and generalization in the language acquisition of children with autism has been reported as a major limitation of using DTT and/or traditional behavioral approaches (Koegel 2000; National Research Council 2001; Wetherby and Woods 2008).

Applied behavioral analysis in communication and language training

ABA is a more broadly based behavioral approach than the traditional DTT approach. Additionally, more extensive research has been conducted on ABA than on DTT approaches. Behavior analysis has already contributed substantially to the treatment of children with autism, and ABA has been utilized with a wide range of autistic behaviors since the

1990s (Paul and Sutherland 2005; Sturmey and Fitzer 2007; Sundberg and Michael 2001). ABA was developed from the work of B.F. Skinner and other behaviorists. ABA approaches demonstrate that every behavior contains three parts: the antecedent (what happens just prior to the behavior occurring), the behavior (what happens after the antecedent has occurred), and the consequence of the behavior (what happens after the behavior has occurred). ABA frequently involves using the information acquired through the functional analysis of antecedents and consequences to interpret the relationship between the behavior and the circumstances in which it appears. The primary emphasis in ABA is the use of direct instructional methods with strong motivational variables (i.e. reinforces, or establishing operation) that alter particular behaviors in systematic and measurable ways. Sturmey and Fitzer (2007) noted that teaching approaches derived from ABA are the most extensively studied interventions for teaching new skills to individuals with ASD. Research indicates that some children benefit much more than others from ABA-based teaching procedures (Sturmey and Fitzer 2007; Sundberg and Michael 2001). ABA is particularly useful for children with ASD in their very early stages of communicative development by increasing responsiveness to language, developing early receptive language concepts, increasing the ability to imitate vocal behavior, eliciting first words and increasing expressive language complexity, increasing symbol play, and decreasing behaviors that interfere with the child's ability to learn from instruction.

Use of music in behavior training for individuals with ASD

ABA has often utilized music, especially songs, in its language assessments and training programs (Barbera 2007; Maurice, Green and Luce 1996; Sundberg and Michael 2001; Sundberg and Partington 1998). The authors of the prominent ABA language training manual *Teaching Language to Children with Autism or Other Developmental Disabilities* stated that one of the simplest types of rudimentary conversation acquired by children is their ability to fill in missing words from songs (Sundberg and Partington 1998). Barbera (2007), the author of *The Verbal Behavior Approach*, reported that, with an ABA verbal behavior approach, a child with autism spends more time working on expressive language skills such as requesting, labeling, and filling in the blanks with songs. ABA practitioners are instructed to teach many simple types of intraverbal behavior using well-known songs and the favorite ones of the learner (Sundberg and Partington 1998).

Numerous studies and instruction in the ABA approach promote the use of songs in their interventions; however, the theoretical justification for the use of music in the approach or the body of valid research on the effect of music on ABA language training is lacking. Previous studies in ABA approaches did not provide the scientific mechanisms for how songs impact the speech and language of children with autism. As a result, those programs or interventions depended on very limited use of music, and children with autism could not experience the broad range of musical interventions. Research is needed to describe the mechanism and strategy of using music in an ABA verbal behavior approach and to explore systematic interventions with music for enhancing communication skills for children with autism. The research should also establish the protocols of music therapy language training in autism within the common training approaches.

An applied behavior analysis verbal behavior approach

Applied behavior analysis in autism treatment

ABA is based on strong and coherent science and extensive empirical research that is the basis for the technologies and procedures used with individuals with ASD. The methodological elements of ABA approaches in autism include functional analysis, task analysis, and the selection and systematic implementation of effective reinforcers. Functional analysis identifies the antecedents and consequences of a behavior and controls the variables that elicit or eliminate the expression of the behavior. Task analysis is used to break down behaviors into their most fundamental steps. The first step is training intensively until a child can produce a behavior in response to the appropriate environmental stimulus with minimal prompting, and it is systematically chained to the next, until the child can produce the entire sequence of steps as a learned behavior. ABA approaches also identify what may be rewarding for each individual by means of empirical observations. These rewards can be utilized to systematically determine schedules in order to manage behaviors. Reinforcement is crucial for establishing and maintaining appropriate behavior and teaching new skills. Arranged reinforcement is necessary in order for many children with ASD to learn specific skills (Sturmey and Fitzer 2007).

The basic intervention programs within ABA consist largely of identifying goals in terms of specific behaviors to be altered in frequency; recording target behaviors; identifying effective forms of reinforcement;

the use of extinction, shaping, and intermittent reinforcement; the development of operant stimulus control, stimulus prompting, and the fading of prompting; and the development of chaining, generalization, rules, imitation, modeling, and other now well-known behavioral procedures (Sundberg and Michael 2001). In addition, ABA approaches require practitioners to determine the function(s) of the behavior. Behaviorists indicate that every behavior has its own function such as seeking attention or escaping from unwanted situations. Children with autism also have main functions for their behaviors; a child may request an item, or ask to be removed from a situation, or may simply seek sensory input. It is important for practitioners or teachers to develop a strategy for each function of the behavior. For example, attention-seeking behaviors should be treated with one set of interventions (e.g. teaching the child how to request things, or give time out from reinforcement) while all behaviors which serve as an escape should be treated in a different way (e.g. teaching the child to be able to ask for a break or help, giving directions or demands involving motor movements, or prompting followed by reinforcement).

Applied behavior analysis: verbal behavior approach

Developing communication and language skills is a major goal for any training program of children with ASD. Such language training consists of the application of the ABA technology described above commonly called verbal behavior. ABA VB has contributed substantially to the treatment of children with autism by gains and results from Skinner's (1957) analysis of language in verbal behavior (Sundberg and Michael 2001). Behavior analysis in general, and Skinner's analysis of verbal behavior in particular, has provided a solid methodology for language assessment and training programs for children with autism based on a large body of empirical research.

VERBAL BEHAVIOR APPROACH

The application of Skinner's behavioral analysis on verbal behavior was developed at Western Michigan University in the 1970s under the direction of Dr Jack Michael. The verbal behavior or applied verbal behavior (AVB) approach not only builds on the science of ABA research, but also enhances a child's ability to learn functional language (Barbera 2007; Sturmey and Fitzer 2007). The VB approach adds ABA to teach all skills, including, most importantly, language skills, to children with autism and related disorders. According to this approach, language is treated as a behavior that can be shaped and reinforced while careful attention is paid to not only what a child is saying but also why he or she is using the language. The VB approach is a fairly new and popular approach that emerged from the basic teachings of ABA, but expands to include B.F. Skinner's analysis of these concepts presented in *Verbal Behavior* (Skinner 1957).

VERBAL BEHAVIOR

Skinner (1957) defined verbal behavior as behavior that is reinforced through the mediation of another person's behavior. Skinner suggested that verbal behavior (i.e. talking) is a learned behavior controlled by environmental variables such as motivation, reinforcement, and antecedent stimuli. He concentrated on the verbal behavior of the individual speaker and referred to the unit of the verbal behavior as a verbal operant, with operant implying a type or class behavior as a distinct form of a particular response instance. He also referred to a set of such units in a particular individual as a verbal repertoire.

VERBAL OPERANTS

Skinner (1957) also distinguished between several different types of verbal operants by its function and defined the elementary verbal operants: mand, tact, echoic (i.e. vocal imitation), intraverbal, textual, transcriptive,[1] and copying a text. According to Skinner (1957), a mand is verbal behavior controlled by a motivational variable (deprivation, satisfaction, or aversive stimulation), and a tact is verbal behavior controlled by a nonverbal stimulus such as a picture, photo, or object. The echoic, intraverbal, textual, copying a text, and transcriptive operants are types of verbal behavior controlled by verbal stimuli. Among Skinner's (1957) functional analysis of verbal behavior, mand, tact, echoic, and intraverbal are exclusively utilized in ABA VB approaches. In terms of its function, mand is a verbal operant of requesting, tact is a verbal operant of labeling or describing, echoic is a verbal operant of vocal imitation, and intraverbal is a verbal operant of social interaction or conversation. By establishing the elementary verbal operants (i.e. mand, tact, echoic, and intraverbal), functional language skills and advanced social communication techniques such as why questions, story telling, picture descriptions, general knowledge questions, and social reciprocation are addressed in the VB approach.

---

1   Transcriptive means that something is transcribed. It indicates a representation in writing of the actual pronunciation of a speech sound, word, or piece of continuous text.

Skinner (1957) viewed the verbal operants as a unit of analysis. He indicated that the same form of verbal response exists in different types of verbal operants; the same word might function differently in different situations. For example, a tendency to say "dog" as a result of hearing someone else say "dog" is echoic behavior, a tendency to say "dog" as a result of seeing an actual dog or a picture of a dog is a tact, and a tendency to say "dog" as a result of seeing the word dog on a chalkboard is a textual behavior. A tendency to say "dog" as a result of hearing someone else say "animal" or sing "there was a farmer who had a _____" is an example of an intraverbal operant, and a tendency to say "dog" to ask to touch a real dog is a mand. Skinner (1957) suggested that the mand *dog*, the tact *dog*, the echoic *dog*, and the intraverbal *dog* involve separate functional relations which can be explained only by discovering all relevant variables. It is concluded that different verbal operants are associated with independent functional control.

This independent functional control is especially important for language training with pre-verbal children who have language impairments (Skinner 1957; Sundberg and Michael 2001). A typically developing child can acquire a functional relation of one form as a tact, for example, and then have it available without further training as a mand, but this kind of spontaneous generalization from one verbal operant to another might be difficult for children with autism who may not have had the adequate exposure to verbal stimuli and other related environment events due to the disorder (Sundberg and Michael 2001). Such training should be based on verbal operant analysis in terms of its function and controlling variables, and the behavior functional unit for the individual speaker and listener should be emphasized.

Use of music in the ABA VA approach

Teaching approaches derived from ABA are the most extensively studied interventions for teaching new skills to children with ASD. Music therapy can be explored for the practice and procedure in developing social communication and language skills in children with autism. Therefore, it is worthwhile to incorporate the ABA VB approach with another effective language training tool, music, in developing new treatment strategies for improving functional language skills and social communication in children with autism. There is a similarity between music and verbal stimuli, and the intact ability to perceive and produce verbal stimuli embedded in or attached to music stimuli in children with autism. Because of its inherent structure, music stimuli can be used as effective antecedent variables and a strong reinforcement in ABA VB language training for children with autism. In particular, music stimuli can be replaced with verbal stimuli in the language training, which is often associated with demands and/or a rigid didactic approach.

Use of music for reinforcement
DEVELOPING REINFORCERS IN THE ABA VA APPROACH

In order to teach language skills to children with ASD, it may first be necessary to get the child to cooperate with the instructor; and the most effective way to increase cooperation is the use of a child's current level of motivation. For example, if the child wants to watch a video, the instructor might use the motivation along with the reinforcement of turning on the video to establish targeted verbal behaviors. The desired training relationship is established when the instructor is consistently associated (paired) with the delivery of reinforcing items and events to the child. Consequently, it is also important that the instructor is not associated with the removal of the items or ongoing reinforcing activities (Sundberg and Partington 1998).

At the beginning of ABA VB language training, it is critical to identify and select powerful idiosyncratic reinforcers for the child. These reinforcers may be consumable (e.g. food, drinks); can easily allow for a short duration of contact (e.g. bubbles, tickles); are relatively easy to remove from the child (e.g. music, video); are easy to deliver (e.g. books, cars, dolls); can be delivered on multiple occasions (e.g. small candies, sips of juice); and always seem strong (e.g. favorite toy, playing outside). Such reinforcers need to be individually chosen for each child, and can be controlled easily and changed daily (Barbera 2007; Sundberg and Partington 1998). Developing age-appropriate reinforcers is as important as determining the most powerful reinforcers for the child, because the language age or developmental age of many children with autism may be different from their chronological age (Lim 2010; Prizant and Wetherby 2005). The process of developing the effective reinforcers for verbal behaviors, and pairing the learning environment, people, or materials with the reinforcements, should be established, since it facilitates designing the curriculum of continuous language training (i.e. selecting target words/ phrases).

Music as reinforcement

The most fundamental principle of the ABA VB approach is to select and use the effective reinforcement for every trial in the training (Barbera 2007; Maurice *et al.* 1996; Paul and Sutherland 2005; Sturmey and Fitzer 2007; Sundberg and Michael 2001; Sundberg and Partington 1998). High preference stimuli are the most likely to function as effective reinforcers (Sturmey and Fitzer 2007). My own research found that music stimuli were more effective for learning and producing functional vocabulary words than speech stimuli for children with ASD (Lim 2010). These children were attentive longer while watching the music video than watching the speech video, even though the music video was longer than the speech video (Lim 2010). The research findings suggest that children with autism have a perceptual preference for and an intact capacity to perceive musical stimuli. Music can be a highly motivating medium for treating language impairment in children with autism.

Musical experience for an establishing operation

Music can function as an establishing operation (EO)[2] in the ABA VB incorporated language training. In particular, various musical experiences can provide children with autism with effective motivational variables (i.e. EO) for many communicative behaviors such as eye contact, pointing, manding, echoic imitation, initiating, entraining, singing, playing instruments, waiting, sharing, receptive language, joint attention, and interaction. Auditory stimuli in musical sounds are commonly used to capture and sustain children's attention (Lim 2010). Various musical instruments and their resultant sounds can motivate children to touch, play, and request the instruments, and create musical sounds. Furthermore, the motivational variables established in such musical experiences result in a natural social interaction between singers or players who share the same musical experiences. Age-appropriate and well-facilitated musical experiences can provide powerful motivational variables and ongoing reinforcing activities for establishing such rapport between peers. In addition, giving the child continuous opportunities to participate and engage in musical experiences functions as a positive reinforcement for appropriate communicative behaviors.

---

2   An establishing operation enables music to set the "mood" naturally for the child to produce the desirable behaviors. EO is a broader term for (automatic) reinforcement and motivation. Music stimuli provide the opportunities to operate verbal production in children with ASD.

MUSIC FOR AUTOMATIC REINFORCEMENT

Music can also function as an automatic reinforcement. Skinner used the term *automatic reinforcement* to indicate that reinforcement occurs without manipulating or demeaning the learner (Sundberg and Michael 2001). Automatic reinforcement involves a strengthening effect that occurs without the deliberate consequential mediation of another person, but rather as a result of an antecedent pairing of a neutral stimulus with an established form of reinforcement (Sundberg, Michael and Partington 1996). Such reinforcement is the result of pairing what the learner needs to learn with what he or she wants as reinforcers, and the paired behavior with reinforcement becomes a target behavior for further training. Use of automatic reinforcement is encouraged in early language training and continues to play an important role in the development of the more complex aspects of verbal behavior.

An example of the application of an automatic reinforcement procedure is pairing a song sung by a music therapist with playing a drum. This particular pairing might increase vocal behavior in a child with autism who enjoys playing the drum and facilitate the development of different verbal operants such as echoic and mand. Playing instruments becomes a strong reinforcer for the child; then singing (verbal behavior) becomes reinforcing. This particular pairing of musical experiences establishes the automatic reinforcement that increases the frequency of verbal behaviors in singing. This automatic reinforcement in a musical activity can address various goals for language training and improve communication skills in children with autism. Sundberg and Michael (2001) noted that language training should be fun for the child and paired with automatic reinforcement as much as possible rather than with the aversive stimuli often associated with demands. Musical experience can provide fun for children, and can therefore automatically reinforce further musical and non-musical behaviors.

Natural environment training

Although a variety of studies have documented the efficacy of didactic approaches (i.e. DTT) and/or traditional ABA approaches in eliciting initial language from previously non-speaking children with autism, these approaches rely heavily on teacher direction, prompted responses, and contrived forms of reinforcement (Koegel 2000; Paul and Sutherland

2005). An inherent weakness in the didactic approach lies in the fact that it often leads to a passive style of communication, in which children respond to prompts to communicate but do not initiate communication or use the verbal behaviors acquired in the training spontaneously to interact with others (Paul and Sutherland 2005). For children with autism to be judged as socially competent during communicative interactions, spontaneous initiations are necessary (Jones, Feeley and Takacs 2007; Koegel 2000). The difficulties in initiating spontaneous verbal behaviors and generalizing and maintaining the behaviors taught through didactic approaches and a few traditional ABA approaches led to the introduction of more naturalistic methods of intervention such as milieu teaching (Paul and Sutherland 2005).

NATURAL ENVIRONMENT IN LANGUAGE TRAINING

Milieu teaching refers to language-teaching methods that are integrated into a child's natural environment (Mancil, Conroy and Haydon 2009; Paul and Sutherland 2005). Milieu teaching approaches include adaptations of behavioral approaches and utilize everyday, natural environments (e.g. home or classroom) for training. Activities take place throughout the day and preferred toys and activities are included in the environment so that participation in activities is self-reinforcing (i.e. automatic reinforcement and EO). In milieu teaching, the child initiates the teaching situation by gesturing or indicating an interest in a desired object or activity and expanded child responses are rewarded with access to the desired object or activity (Paul and Sutherland 2005). Delprato (2001) reported that naturalistic language training combined with the milieu teaching methods is more effective than discrete-trial training for young children with autism.

Many ABA practitioners have adopted naturalistic methods in which instructional episodes are initiated by the child's behavior toward objects the teacher plants in the environment; instruction takes place in the context of natural activities, using objects of high interest to the child. To operate within the framework of contemporary ABA, the child selects the stimuli from a range provided by the teacher, and the teacher delivers prompts based upon the child's initiating behavior, rather than in a prescribed fashion (Koegel 2000; Paul and Sutherland 2005; Prizant and Wetherby 2005; Shafer 1994; Sundberg and Partington 1998). The combination of these approaches may improve spontaneous interaction and the generalization of new behaviors in children with autism.

MUSIC FOR NATURAL ENVIRONMENT TRAINING

Use of music can make an integrative bridge between naturalistic approaches (i.e. milieu teaching) and the didactic ABA VB approaches. Systemically designed music activities establish automatic reinforcement and preferred experiences for children. Music time in the classroom establishes the natural environment for children with autism and provides the necessary structure for the language training. Various musical instruments and favorite songs are used as motivational variables and natural reinforcers. An active music-making experience with these instruments and songs increases spontaneous communication with adults and peers (Adamek, Thaut and Furman 2008; Lim 2010). The child initiates the teaching situation by creating musical sounds or leading an improvisational ensemble. Group music therapy interventions in the child's natural environments can provide him or her with ample opportunities to practice communication skills such as responding to others, holding hands with a peer, singing along, taking turns, listening, sharing ideas, greeting others, and sharing instruments and equipment. Musical interventions facilitated by parents or caregivers in a child's home also establish a natural learning environment for him or her. The instructor can establish musical contact and set up ensuing musical interaction that requires daily functional communication and social interaction such as imitation, call and response, and improvisation.

Language assessment in the ABA VB approach with music

Considering language as an interaction between speakers and listeners with the verbal operants as the basic functional units implies the relevance of these units for an assessment of language deficits in autism (Sundberg and Michael 2001). The primary purpose of a language assessment in ABA VB music therapy is to identify specific verbal deficits and to serve as a guide for the development of an appropriate language intervention program for the individual being assessed (Sundberg and Partington 1998). The assessment may require materials such as well-known children's songs, a collection of objects, musical instruments, pictures or photos, and common reinforcers (e.g. cookie, toy, or sticker). ABA VB starts the language assessment by obtaining information about the child's mand repertoire (Barbera 2007; Shafer 1994; Sundberg and Michael 2001).

Mand assessment with music

Mand is a type of language in which the form of the child's verbal response is controlled by what the child requests or by a motivational variable (i.e. EO). Thus, the purpose of assessing mand is to determine how the child presents his or her needs and desires (Sundberg and Partington 1998). Many children acquire this verbal skill quite quickly with little instruction; however, children with autism may have deficits in learning how to use words to ask for what they want. According to the VB approach, a vocabulary word is not a mand if there is no motivation preceding it. Therefore, a mand must receive reinforcement specific to that particular mand; while the other verbal operants (echoic, tact, intraverbal) typically receive nonspecific reinforcement, including some form of generalized conditioned reinforcement such as social attention, approval, or termination of a demand (Sundberg and Michael 2001). As a result, a mand directly and immediately benefits the speaker by producing access to desired reinforcers.

For example, if a child wants a cookie, he or she asks for it. Skinner (1957) indicated that motivation is often precipitated by satiation and deprivation. If a child loves cookies (i.e. motivational variable or establishing operation) and mands for them and receives them, the child will eventually satisfy his or her desire for a cookie (after eating his or her fill of cookies) and will then mand for water or juice. The desire must come prior to the mand. Therefore, in order to assess manding skills, it is recommended to select anything which is out of sight that the child currently requests without a prompt. For example, the teacher presents a small piece of cookie and sees if the child takes it and eats it. If the child does, the child's motivation is strong, and the teacher holds up another piece of cookie. At this time, the teacher waits five seconds to see if the child says or signs the word (Barbera 2007; Sundberg and Partington 1998).

In order to assess mand with music stimuli, the music therapist must determine musical sounds that the child prefers; this information can be obtained from the child and/or his or her parents or teachers. Based on the information that the child enjoys guitar sounds, the music therapist plays the guitar for ten seconds and stops playing. If the child reaches or touches the guitar, his or her motivation is strong to continue to hear or play the guitar. The music therapist starts playing the guitar again and stops. At this time, the music therapist waits for five seconds to see if the child says "guitar" or a word for requesting more playing.

Echoic assessment with music

The echoic operant involves repeating what someone else says, similar to an echo. A child's ability to repeat sounds and words (i.e. echoic behavior) plays a very important role in language acquisition and speech development (Lim 2010; Prizant and Wetherby 1993; Sundberg and Partington 1998; Tager-Flusberg 1985). Information regarding the quality and strength of the echoic repertoire from vocal imitation can reveal potential problems in producing response topographies that are essential for other verbal interactions. If the child cannot echo specific sounds, then the probability of those responses occurring in other functional units of verbal behavior is quite low (Lim 2010; Prizant and Wetherby 1993, 2005; Sundberg and Michael 2001; Tager-Flusberg 1985). If a nonverbal child cannot repeat any sounds or words, the child may be a candidate for the use of sign language or non-speech augmentative communication devices. To assess a child's echoic skills, no materials or items should be present, and the child should be sitting near the evaluator. Simple sounds such as "Say ma" and "Say ba" need to be assessed first; if the child echoes simple sounds, one-syllable words such as "Say cup" and "Say ball" are used. The echoic assessment should move forward to assess multisyllable words and then phrases (Barbera 2007). During the assessment, a child who has a strong vocal imitation repertoire may be able to learn these skills quickly given the appropriate teaching procedures, even though still unable to ask for reinforcers or to label items in the environment (Sundberg and Partington 1998).

To assess a child's echoic skills, simple sounds with a definite pitch or rhythmic figure such as "Sing ma (E)" and "Say ba ba (♫)" should be implemented first. If the child echoes simple combinations of musical patterns, the next step is to sing simple melodies and rhythms with several different (adjacent) pitches such as "Sing (C) La (D) La (B) La (C)" and "Sing (C) Ya (G) Woo (E) Ya (F) Woo (D) Ya (E) Woo (C)." The echoic assessment should move forward to assess singing entire phrases with actual words.

Tact assessment with music

Tact is the ability to verbally label common items that a child can see, smell, taste, hear, touch, and feel. A tact is associated with the meaning of the vocabulary word; however, this skill is different from the receptive identification of items or actions. Tacting is a more difficult skill because the child must not only identify the correct word, but also be able to have the vocal control to independently pronounce the word (Sundberg and Partington 1998). To assess a child's tact skills, photos of the child's favorite reinforcers and the instructor's verbal request to tact (i.e. label) the items are used. The actual items can be used in the tact assessment; however, this may cause confusion between manding for the item and tacting (Barbera 2007). A more advanced tacting ability can be assessed with objects, flash cards, and pictures (from magazines) by asking the child "What is it?" and recording the child's responses. A strong ability to tact items and actions can be seen in a child who easily and quickly acquires new vocabulary words and retains those words without intensive training (Sundberg and Partington 1998).

In order to assess tact with music, the music therapist prepares pictures or photos of the child's favorite instruments. The music therapist plays a small drum and asks "What is this?" or presents photos or pictures of a drum and asks the child to tact (i.e. label) the items. If the child says "drum," the therapist gives the child the drum to play.

Intraverbal assessment with music

A systematic examination of the receptive language and intraverbal repertoires can predict the child's ability to process various verbal stimuli. Many children with autism show difficulty in answering questions and participating in meaningful conversations, despite having the ability to speak hundreds of vocabulary words. Conversational skills consist of intraverbal behaviors which are important for social interaction, as well as for the acquisition of academic skills. Intraverbal behaviors are clearly a type of language skill that is different from requesting reinforcers (i.e. mand), and from labeling objects, actions, adjectives, etc. (i.e. tact). One of the simplest ways to assess a child's intraverbal skill is to ask the child to complete words from familiar phrases. The key to assessing this skill is to speak a phrase that the child has heard many times and then to leave out the last word of each line. For example, when reading a story book, the evaluator begins by reading slowly aloud "Brown bear, brown bear, what do you _____?" and leaves the final word off. If the child does not fill in the word "see," then the evaluator says it, and goes on the next line, "I see the yellow duck looking at _____," waiting a few seconds for the child to fill in the word "me."

If the child is able to fill in one-word blanks in familiar phrases, the next step in assessing the intraverbal skill is to ask the child to fill in more functional phrases by saying "You sleep in a _____" or "You drink from a _____." If the child can fill in "bed" and "cup," the evaluator might ask more complex intraverbals such as "What flies in the sky?" "Where are you going?" or "What fruit is yellow?" (Barbera 2007; Sundberg and Partington 1998). Children who can easily answer a number of specific questions, with obvious variation in their answers, might begin to demonstrate emerging conversational skills.

Intraverbal assessment starts with the child's favorite song; this information can be obtained from parents or teachers of the child. If the child enjoys watching *Barney*, the music therapist plays the guitar and sings loudly and slowly "I love _____" and leaves the final word off. If the child does not fill in the word "you," the music therapist sings it while playing the proper chord on the guitar, and goes on the next line, "You love _____," waiting a few seconds for the child to fill in the word "me." This particular technique of language acquisition is called filling in missing words from songs and utilizes a common Gestalt law of perception (i.e. the law of good continuation), which involves perceptual completion (Lim 2010). The target word in a song placed at the end of each phrase allows the child to anticipate the location and time of the target words to be produced. The structurally and functionally organized singing experience enhances speech production and vocabulary acquisition in children with ASD.

The fundamental verbal operants assessed for further language training in the ABA VB approach include mand, echoic, tact, and intraverbal. The ABA VB approach commonly assesses other communication skills such as motor imitation, vocal play, sample matching (i.e. ability to match pictures, designs, and shapes to identical samples), receptive language (i.e. ability to understand and act upon specific words and phrases), identification of letters and numbers, and social interaction (Barbera 2007; Sundberg and Partington 1998). The presented language assessment with music is designed to reflect the average performance of typical two- or three-year-old children (Sundberg and Michael 2001). Listening to guitar sounds, singing a short melody, and playing the drum can be used as a reinforcement for the assessment. In addition, the antecedent stimuli in language assessment may include both verbal and musical stimuli (i.e. guitar accompaniment). The music therapist can also assess the child's motor imitation by singing "head and shoulder" and pointing to the body parts. Receptive language skills can be assessed by saying "Play your drum fast" or "Play your drum three times."

Language training in the ABA VB approach with music

Language training: verbal operants training in DSLM

A music therapy session consists of numerous trials for various verbal operants (i.e. mand, echoic, tact, and intraverbal) and transferring trials across the different verbal operants. At the beginning of the music therapy treatment, a one-to-one setting is appropriate for teaching each verbal operant. As the child becomes familiar with the structure of the music therapy protocols and repertoire, the verbal operants can be combined and social interaction should be included in the language training (Paul and Sutherland 2005; Sundberg and Partington 1998). Group music therapy is strongly recommended for the children who have mastered the basic verbal operants training but still need to practice spontaneous initiation in communication and social interaction with peers. The combination of individual and group music therapy can be an effective model for language training for children with autism. It is also important to generalize the training procedures from a specific training session to the child's natural environment.

The use of music in speech and language training for children with ASD should address the following strategies:

- recognizing the importance of music for the children's learning, development, and socio-cultural participation

- adapting to each child's unique interests, musical preference, developmental levels, and learning style

- identifying the function of musical stimuli and analyzing each child's musical responses

- identifying and selecting the musical stimulus or musical experience which is intrinsically motivating for the child

- creating and supporting opportunities that include typically developing peers as musical partners

- being open and creative to reach each child's full potential for the music-making experience.

This section includes mechanisms and techniques of music therapy language training incorporated within the ABA VB approach. The examples and strategies suggested below are designed for preschoolers (age range three to five years) with language deficits due to autism.

Mand training in DSLM

From the perspective of Skinner's functional analysis of verbal behavior, it is reasonable for mand training to be the major focus of early language training (Shafer 1994; Sundberg and Michael 2001). Many young children with autism have no tendency to request objects or items that they obviously want, which indicates that they do not use language to control their environment for their own benefit. Objects could be used as an effective form of reinforcement for the children, and the ability to verbally request the reinforcers allows them to control their environment. Not only do mands allow a child to control the delivery of conditioned and unconditioned reinforcers, but also they begin to establish the speaker and listener roles that are essential for further verbal development. Mands are also the most likely type of verbal behavior to be emitted spontaneously, and the generalization may occur quickly because of the unique effects of the motivational reinforcer or EO (Sundberg and Michael 2001). Other types of verbal behavior should not be neglected; but the child may gain control over the social and the non-social environment by the mands. This control should increase the value of language training in general, responsiveness to language, and the ability to initiate first words. Mands are also the type of VB to be emitted spontaneously, and the generalization may occur quickly because of the unique effects of the motivational reinforcer or EO (Sundberg and Michael 2001). For more detail about Mand training see pages 106–110.

Advanced mand training

Sundberg and Michael (2001) suggested a few fundamental techniques for advanced mand training in the ABA VB approach. First, in order to teach mands of missing items, mand training should occur in the absence of the object or condition that is the reinforcement for the mand with a question such as "What do you look for?" Second, in mand training for information, questions can be mands that are reinforced by verbal behavior on the part of the listener. The value of the information defines the motivational variables and the level of reinforcement (Sundberg *et al.* 2002). The EO begins with teaching a child to say "Where is the cup?" (i.e. mand) as an echoic response and then providing the information "On the table" (i.e. specific reinforcement). The most relevant and specific EO must be present during this type of mand training. Last, mands to remove aversive stimuli can be trained. Children with autism need to be specifically taught to say each of the mands (e.g. "go away," "don't," "stop," "give that back," "leave me alone"). In this particular type of mand training, the aversive stimulus must be present during training, and terminating the aversive stimulus must be the main form of reinforcement for the correct response (Sundberg and Michael 2001). The specific use of the EO is an independent variable in mand training, and it can also be used as an additional independent variable for echoic, tact, and intraverbal training. A successful mand training program implemented by the EO can facilitate the later development of other verbal behaviors and communication skills.

Example: DSLM mand training[3]

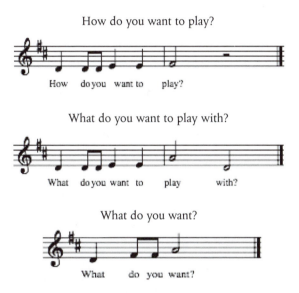

How do you want to play?

What do you want to play with?

What do you want?

Echoic training in DSLM

The ultimate goal of echoic training is to increase the child's spontaneous use of speech, and to bring specific vocalization (i.e. verbalization) under imitative control (Sundberg and Partington 1998). The first procedure in echoic training involves the use of direct reinforcement for any vocalization or verbalization of the child, so that the frequency of the

---

3   The music and lyrics in each of the examples in this chapter are by Hayoung A. Lim and Ellary Draper.

verbal production and reinforcement might be increased. One technique for increasing the verbal production is to pair the instructor's vocalizations (e.g. "bounce, bounce") with naturally occurring reinforcers such as bouncing the child on the ball. Sounds can be used as reinforcers to modify the child's behavior. In such cases it is possible for these sounds to become automatically strengthened (paired with fun) for the child to produce. Skinner (1957) identified this effect as "automatic reinforcement" to indicate that the reinforcement occurred as the automatic result of the response (Sundberg and Michael 2001; Sundberg and Partington 1998). Such reinforcement automatically increases the frequency of the verbal behavior and facilitates the development of echoic and mand (Sundberg and Michael 2001). For more detail about echoic training see pages 119–121.

Example: DSLM echoic training

Good morning, good morning. (Name) says good morning.

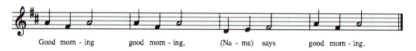

I want more, I want more, can you say "I want more"?

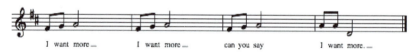

Mommy says I love you. (Name) says I love you.

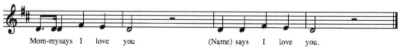

Nice to meet you, nice to meet you, can you say "nice to meet you"?

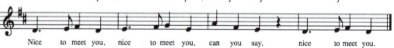

It's time to go, it's time to go. I say see you later, you say see you later.

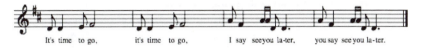

Have a good day, have a good day, can you say "have a good day"?

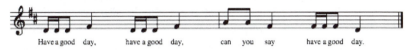

Tact training in DSLM

Tact training can begin with presenting a nonverbal stimulus and requesting speech as the response. The antecedent for a tact is some form of nonverbal stimulus (e.g. the actual item, a picture, a sound, or a smell), and the consequence for a tact is nonspecific reinforcement, such as praise. Technically, the antecedent for a pure tact will not include any verbal stimulus or instructor's question (e.g. "What is it?" "What do you hear?"); however, it is almost impossible to teach tacting without asking such questions. Therefore, in the ABA VB approach, tact training will include both the nonverbal stimulus and a question from the instructor (Barbera 2007). Tact training might begin with the same words that were used for mand training and expand to the new words. Children with autism learn to ask for items they want fairly quickly because it results in their getting those items; however, it is also important for the children to be able to identify those items even when they do not want the item or the item itself is not forthcoming. In tact training, the children are reinforced with praise or some other item or event for being correct in their labeling of the item, but the children do not receive the item that they had previously learned to request. In order to teach a tact, it is necessary to transfer that verbal response from the control of the motivational variable to the control of the nonverbal item itself and to other nonspecific reinforcements such as praise or favorite activities.

The initial tact training in music therapy should also begin with antecedent variables including motivational variables (EO), a verbal stimulus to respond, a nonverbal stimulus, and an echoic stimulus. If the target response is "drum," the child should strongly want a drum (i.e. EO), and the desired item, a drum (i.e. nonverbal stimulus), should be present. The procedure for actual tact training begins when the instructor starts to phase out the echoic prompt ("Say drum"), while keeping in the verbal stimulus "What is it?" The verbal stimulus should also be continuously reduced until the child's response "drum" occurs in the absence of the verbal prompts. The child needs to learn to spontaneously identify at least some objects or pictures without being verbally prompted.

The next step of the tact training is to phase out the elements of the mand (i.e. the delivery of the drum) and to transfer control from motivation to the nonverbal item itself by changing from a specific reinforcement (a drum) to a nonspecific reinforcement (e.g. praise or sticker). In addition, the verbal stimuli "What is it?" versus "What do you want to play?" can help the child to discriminate between the two separate conditions of mand and tact (Sundberg and Partington 1998). This particular procedure might be effectively established when the instructor uses a picture of a drum rather than a real drum. The last step consists of a spontaneous verbal response controlled only by a nonverbal stimulus and nonspecific reinforcement. For example, the child looks at a picture of a drum or a real drum and says "drum" without any verbal prompts. Tact training with pictures will eventually increase the number of vocabulary words produced by children with autism. The tact repertoire can also be enhanced by increasing the complexity of the response by including more words to describe events in the environment (Lim 2010; Sundberg and Partington 1998).

The procedure for actual tact training begins when the instructor starts to phase out the echoic prompt ("Say drum"), while keeping in the verbal stimulus "What is it?" The verbal stimulus should also be continuously reduced until the child's response "drum" occurs in the absence of the verbal prompts. The child needs to learn to spontaneously identify at least some objects or pictures without being verbally prompted. The last step of tact training consists of a spontaneous verbal response controlled only by a nonverbal stimulus and nonspecific reinforcement. For example, the child looks at a picture of a drum or a real drum and says "drum" without any verbal prompts (Sundberg and Partington 1998). Tact training with pictures will eventually increase the number of vocabulary words produced by children with autism (Lim 2010). The tact repertoire can also be enhanced by increasing the complexity of the response by including more words to describe events in the environment (Sundberg and Partington 1998). In addition, tact training can be further developed to teach letters, numbers, and other pre-academic skills to the children.

It is important to begin tact training with the words that the child has already produced in mand or echoic training. If the child shows an ability to mand and imitate (i.e. echoic), the music therapist can start to teach tact skills. In tact training, the music therapist should provide the verbal stimuli (i.e. antecedent variable) with carefully organized musical patterns. The music therapist composes a short melody for the question (i.e. verbal stimuli) such as "What is this? Please tell me. This is _____" or "Can you tell me what this is, what this is?" It is important to start tact training with the words that the child has already produced in mand or echoic training. If the child is able to produce "drum" and "guitar," the music therapist holds up the picture or photo of the drum and guitar and then sings the question. If the child says "drum" and "guitar," the music therapist gives social or musical reinforcement (i.e. nonspecific reinforcement) such as a praise song or hi-five song.

In order to teach a new tact skill, the music therapist uses elements of echoic training and then transfers the verbal operant to a tact. For example, the music therapist sings "*This is a carrot, this is a carrot, carrot*" or "*This is a train, train, train*" with a well-composed melody (considering prosody of the word) while pointing to pictures or photos of the items (e.g. a carrot or a train), and then asks the child to repeat the therapist's singing (i.e. echoic training). If the child can imitate the word in singing, the music therapist holds a picture of an item and sings "*What is this?*" with a prompt (if it is needed). "*This is a* _____." If the child says "carrot" or "train," he or she receives social and/or musical praises (i.e. tacting). This transferring verbal operants training technique (from echoing to tacting) with singing can be used in teaching letters, numbers, and reading skills (e.g. "This is a cup, cup with the letter C" or "This is number seven").

Example: DSLM tact training

What is this? What is this? Can you tell me what this is?

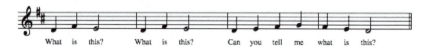

Pink pig. Orange lion. Black cat.

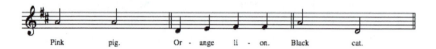

Blue fish. White sheep. Brown horse.

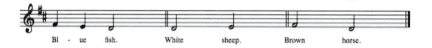

Intraverbal training in DSLM

Intraverbal behavior is a type of expressive language where a word or phrase evokes another word or phrase, but the two are not identical. Intraverbal behavior also consists of word association, such as a tendency to say "mouse" when someone says "Mickey," and responses to fill-in-the-blank items. The intraverbal training is different from the motivational control (EO) of the mand training and the nonverbal control of the tact training in that the verbal responses are controlled by non-matching verbal stimuli (Sundberg and Partington 1998).

Intraverbal training begins with the development of the intraverbal repertoire (Sundberg and Michael 2001; Sundberg and Partington 1998). Such a repertoire prepares a child to produce verbal behavior rapidly and accurately (i.e. pragmatic skills) with respect to further stimulation at a more advanced level, and to make a conversation (Sundberg and Michael 2001). In early intraverbal training, the focus should be on establishing the child's ability to respond intraverbally to the other's verbal behavior using whatever interests the child, even though the verbal responses might be meaningless or less associative. Sundberg and Partington (1998) suggested using the fill-in-the-blank intraverbal repertoire which is directly relevant to the child's ongoing interests and contains words the child hears in the daily environment. This intraverbal repertoire might include not only songs, but also rhymes (e.g. "One, two, buckle my _____"), commonly heard and spoken phrases (e.g. "I love _____"), animal sounds (e.g. "The kitty says _____"), object sounds (e.g. "The train goes _____"), common associations (e.g. "Mommy and _____"), and specific daily activities (e.g. "Put on your shoes and _____") (Barbera 2007; Sundberg and Partington 1998).

Similar to other verbal behavior training, the initial intraverbal training also begins with the antecedent variables including motivational variables (i.e. EO), a verbal stimulus to respond, a nonverbal stimulus, and an echoic stimulus. If the target response is "cracker," the child should strongly want to eat a cracker (i.e. EO), and the desired item, a cracker (i.e. nonverbal stimulus), should be present. The initial trial for intraverbal training will consist of the instructor holding up or pointing to the item (nonverbal stimulus) and saying to the child "You eat a _____" (i.e. verbal stimulus to respond), and/or "Say cracker" (i.e. echoic stimulus). The sample prompting and fading procedures that were described for mand and tact training can be used for intraverbal training (Sundberg and Partington 1998). For a child who can easily mand and tact "cracker," the next trial in the intraverbal training consists of removing the nonverbal stimulus (i.e. cracker) and repeating the verbal stimulus ("You eat a _____"). The instructor should wait several seconds for a correct response and reinforce the correct response with nonspecific reinforcers such as praise, social interaction (e.g. hi-five), or stickers.

Typical children acquire much of their intraverbal repertoire as a result of massive exposure to a complex and rich verbal environment (Sundberg and Michael 2001). However, children with autism who are not strongly reinforced by stimuli in a typical social environment need intensive intraverbal training with extra repertoire. Verbal behavioral analysts and researchers suggest that intraverbal training procedures should be conducted simultaneously with the training of other verbal behaviors including mands, echoics, and tacts (Barbera 2007; Sundberg and Michael 2001; Sundberg and Partington 1998). Effective intraverbal training consists of verbal responses which are already in the child's repertoire as an echoic, mand, or tact (Sundberg and Partington 1998). The intraverbal repertoire for children with autism should be selected from the list of acquired echoics, mands, and tacts, and these words should be utilized under the intraverbal control.

The key strategy in intraverbal training is building an intraverbal repertoire with functional vocabulary words and/or phrases used in daily dialogue. As the child develops an intraverbal repertoire, the music therapist can use pictures or photos of the repertoire as visual prompts and facilitate tact training to intraverbal transfer. This particular music therapy technique called developmental speech and language training through music is designed to utilize musical (i.e. singing) as well as related materials (i.e. pictures) to enhance and facilitate tact and intraverbal operants in children with ASD (Lim 2010; Thaut 2005). The music therapist should compose songs including the target words/phrases which are located at the end of each lyric line. For example, "Look at the *pink pig*. He's wearing *shoes*. Oh, where will you *go*? I'm going to see the *baby*. I will give him a big *hug*. Babies are so much *fun*" (Lim 2010). These songs should be composed in a simple song structure and melodies within a limited pitch range, adjacent intervals, and repetitive melodic contour. The arrangement of musical elements within the song should be developmentally appropriate and syllabic production of the target words/ phrases should be emphasized by the rhythm and harmonic structure as needed to preserve prosody and speech rhythm (Lim 2010). Pictures for each target word/phrase should be presented by the music therapist as she sings the congruent target word/phrase for the tact training. Repetition of the musical and visual presentation can improve the intraverbal skills with modified tacting skills (Lim 2010).

Example: DSLM intraverbal training

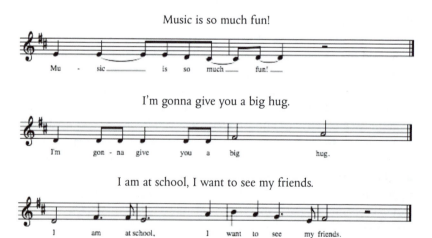

I am hungry, I am hungry, I like to eat.

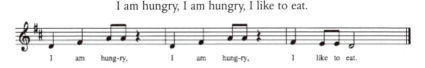

(Name) can sing and play, (name) is happy.

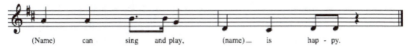

Where is the butterfly, can you point?

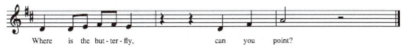

Transfer of the verbal operants

Skinner (1957) indicated in his analysis of *Verbal Behavior* that the same verbal response can occur for different reasons or meanings; these reasons or meanings require different types of control (i.e. echoic, mand, tact, intraverbal, or written). Further, all the meanings need to be taught to the child (Sundberg and Partington 1998). Therefore, separate training for each verbal operant is essential in ABA VB language training, as the child develops more functional language skills; however, it is almost impossible to teach and use only a single verbal operant. Transferring verbal operants in the language training becomes necessary. All of the training procedures described above also involve a transference of procedures: the transferring of stimulus control from a prompted trial to a trial with diminished prompts, to no prompt at all (Barbera 2007). In addition, each tact, echoic, and intraverbal training starts with a mand and transfers it to the desired verbal operant (Sundberg and Partington 1998). Various transfer trials can be used in the VB language training. For example, a tact can be transferred from a echoic: the instructor says "Say ball" and the child says "ball" (echoic) and then the instructor holds up a picture of a ball and says "What is it?" and the child says "ball" (tact). An intraverbal can be produced by a transferred tact: the instructor asks "What number is this?" while holding up the number nine on a flash card, and the child says "nine" (tact); then the instructor asks "How old are you?" when phasing out the visual stimuli, and the child says "nine" (intraverbal). The transfer trials procedures across verbal operants are effective methods for building on the child's strengths in speech and improving functional communication skills (Barbera 2007).

Use of a picture schedule in music therapy language training

It is common to use a schedule in language training for children with autism. Presenting and informing the entire schedule for a session prior to and/or during the session may help the children to sustain their attention and anticipate upcoming experiences. Knowing what is coming next can provide a sense of perceptual safety and confidence for the children. Since most preschoolers with autism have rarely acquired reading skills, using pictures with a schedule board might be appropriate. Pictures for the music therapy session schedule can be obtained from photos of activities, instruments, and simplified illustrations. The Picture Exchange Communication System (Frost and Bondy 1994) has provided numerous pictures for augmenting communication in children with autism (Sundberg and Partington 1998).

Conclusion

Music can be used as a primary tool in the ABA VB language assessment and training interventions for treating the communication deficits of ASD. Music stimuli including various musical instruments and musical sounds can function as antecedent variables in the ABA VB approach including motivational variables (EO), automatic reinforcement, a verbal stimulus to respond, and a nonverbal stimulus in teaching the verbal operants. Pairing target verbal behavior with musical experiences establishes effective automatic reinforcement, and it can increase the frequency of the communicative behaviors and social interaction in children with autism. Participating in ongoing musical activities is a positive reinforcement for continuing the desirable verbal behaviors in children with autism.

Musical behaviors function as target verbal behaviors for the training including mand (i.e. request for musical experience), tact (i.e. naming instruments or musical production and singing with pictures or books), echoic (i.e. singing along and musical imitation), intraverbal (i.e. completing songs, and call and response), and advanced social interaction (i.e. turn-taking and ensemble). Verbal stimuli or prompts for different verbal operants can be embedded in musical stimuli (within a structure of songs), and used by the children to perceive the verbal stimuli attentively and to produce the verbal operants easily. In addition, carefully designed training trials with music experiences facilitate the transfer of the verbal operants and enhance more functional verbal communication and social interaction. Sharing music experiences with peers or adults provides a natural learning environment, in which children with autism develop spontaneous initiations for social interaction and connect the learning experiences into their daily life experiences (i.e. generalization).

Appendix A

Example of Songs for DSLM

1. Hello, hello, *brown bear*

   What do you like to *eat?*

   I like to eat *apples.*

   When I eat apples, I am *happy.*

   Brown bear says, "I want *more.*"

   Daddy bear says, "The apples are *all gone.*"

Song #1

**Music and Words by
Hayoung Audrey Lim**

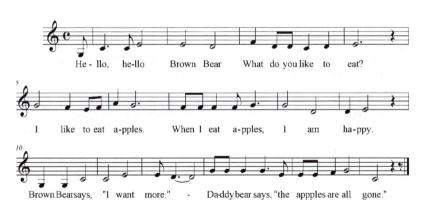

2. In the morning, a yellow duck likes to *play*.

A red bird likes to *sing*.

Oh, the bird sounds so *pretty*.

A green frog says "*Stop.*"

It's time to go *home*.

Everybody says, "I want to see *mommy*."

Song #2

**Music and Words by
Hayoung Audrey Lim**

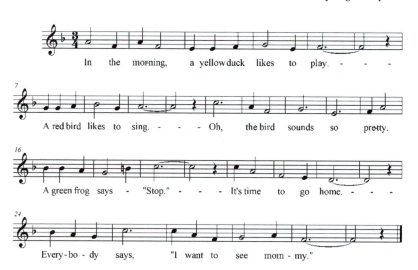

3. Look at the *pink pig*.

   He's wearing *shoes*.

   Oh, where will you *go*?

   I'm going to see the *baby*.

   I'll give him a big *hug*.

   Babies are so much *fun*.

Song #3

Music and Words by
Hayoung Audrey Lim

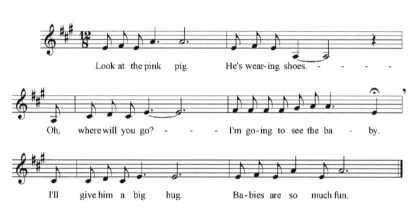

Look at the pink pig. He's wear-ing shoes. - - - -

Oh, where will you go? - - - I'm go-ing to see the ba - by.

I'll give him a big hug. Ba-bies are so much fun.

4. On a starry night, a little boy is running *down*.

    The little boy says, "Hey, *look*!

    I see a butterfly. Can you *point*?

    The butterfly will give you a *kiss*,

    But only when you *sleep*.

    The butterfly will come *again*."

Song #4

Music and Word by
Hayoung Audrey Lim

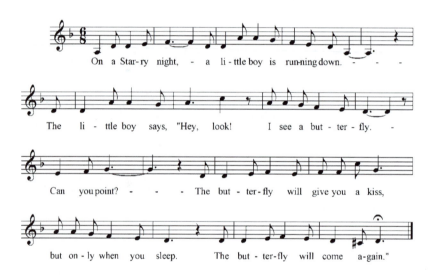

5. Hello, everyone. Let me tell you my *story*.

    One day, I went to the *school*.

    But I couldn't find my *key*.

    My teacher said, "*Come on!*

    Your key is *here*."

    I said, "Thank you, teacher." My story is *all done*.

Song #5

**Music and Words by
Hayoung Audrey Lim**

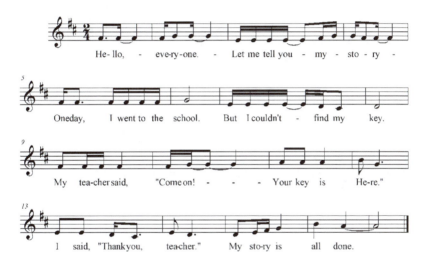

6.   Hey, Mister Monkey, can you come *out*?

"Hi, my friends, I want to say '*Yes.*'

But, I'm busy now. I'm peeling my yellow *banana.*"

Do you know, your hands are *dirty*?

Mister Monkey says, "I know. That's not *okay.*

I think I need a little *help.*"

Song #6

**Music and Words by
Hayoung Audrey Lim**

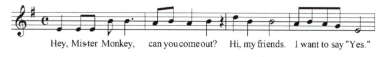

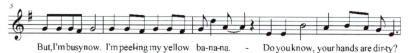

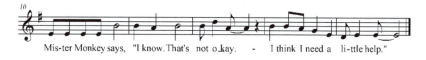

Appendix B

Example of Visual Illustrations for DSLM[1]

Song #1

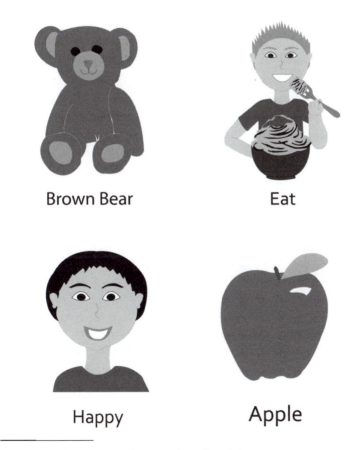

Brown Bear

Eat

Happy

Apple

1   Illustrated by Hayoung Audrey Lim and Jennifer Budnik.

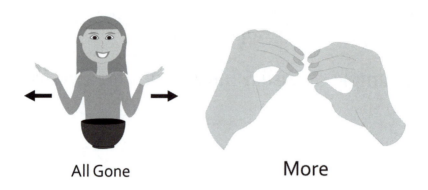

All Gone   More

Song #2

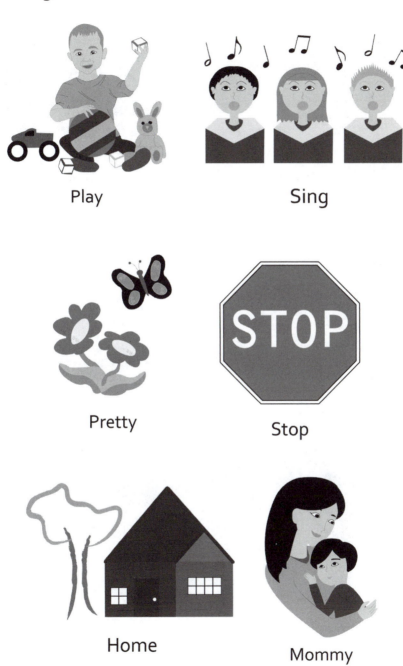

Play

Sing

Pretty

Stop

Home

Mommy

Song #3

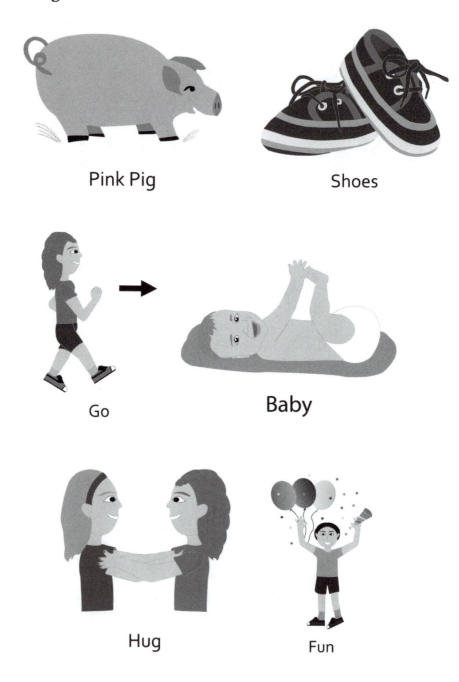

Pink Pig

Shoes

Go

Baby

Hug

Fun

Song #4

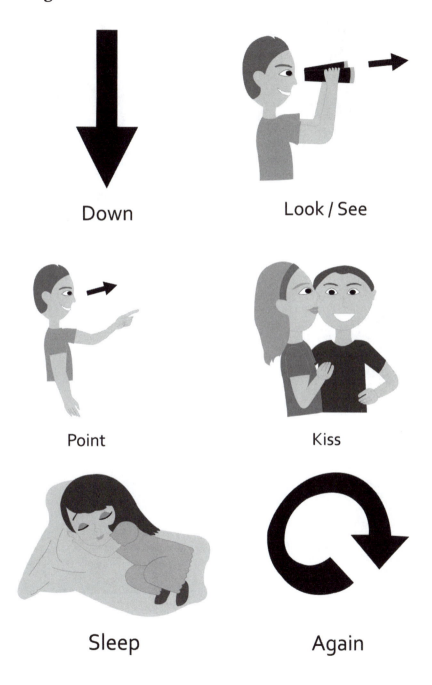

Song #5

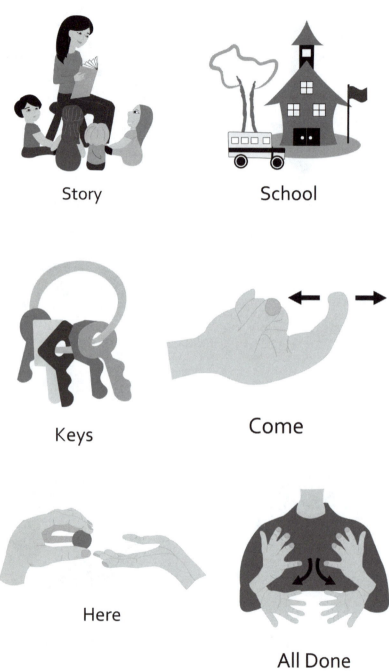

Story

School

Keys

Come

Here

All Done

Song #6

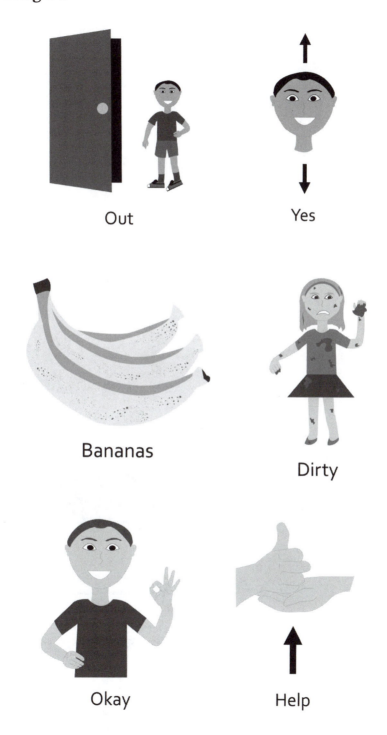

Out

Yes

Bananas

Dirty

Okay

Help

Appendix C

The Effect of Developmental Speech and Language Training through Music on Speech Production in Children with ASD

Introduction

This appendix briefly describes the method and procedure of my original study and reports the results obtained from data collection. It discusses the descriptive and the inferential results from the statistical analysis according to the following four research questions:

1. Does level of speech production in children with ASD differ by training conditions: music versus speech versus no-training?

2. Does level of speech production in children with ASD differ by level of functioning, language age, or presence of echolalia?

3. Does any interaction exist between type of training condition, level of functioning, language age, presence of echolalia, and overall speech production in children with ASD?

4. Does any relationship exist between training conditions: music versus speech and various aspects of speech production, including semantics, phonology, pragmatics, and prosody, in children with ASD?

Much of the practical information about the research study can be found in the main text. For a full account see Lim (2010).

Participants

Fifty-one children were recruited from various local treatment facilities for children with ASD, and a total of fifty children were selected to participate in this study. One child was screened with her parents' consent; however, the child did not participate in the study because she had a dual diagnosis of ASD and Down syndrome. Each child had already been diagnosed with ASD by his or her own health care provider, such as a pediatric psychologist or neurologist. All children met the diagnostic criteria for autism, including qualitative impairments in social functioning and communication, and repetitive behaviors and interests (American Psychiatric Association (APA) 1994). Each child displayed the four central characteristics of ASD, including: (1) disturbances of language and communication, (2) ritualistic and compulsive behaviors and insistence on sameness, (3) disturbed social relationships, and (4) onset of the disorder prior to 30 months of age (Kanner 1946; Paul and Sutherland 2005; Prizant and Duchan 1981; Tager-Flusberg 1997). Table A.1 gives the demographic information of the participants' age, level of functioning, language age, echolalia, and gender.

Table A.1 Participants' age, level of functioning, language age, echolalia, and gender

	Music	Speech	No-training
Number of participants (N=50)	18	18	14
Age range			
3 years (N=6)	2	2	2
4 years (N=20)	6	7	7
5 years (N=24)	10	9	5
Level of functioning			
High (N=25)	8	12	5
Low (N=25)	10	6	9

Language age and characteristics			
1 year (N=9)	2	2	5
1.5 years (N=5)	1	2	2
2 years (N=6)	5	0	1
2.5 years (N=7)	2	4	1
3 years (N=5)	2	2	1
3.5 years (N=8)	4	3	1
4 years (N=10)	2	5	3
Echolalia			
Presence (N=32)	13	12	7
Absence (N=18)	5	6	7
Gender			
Girls (N=6)	3	2	1
Boys (N=44)	15	16	13

Materials

Target words/phrases were selected from functional vocabularies that typically developing children can use effectively in everyday interactions (Prizant *et al.* 1997; Sundberg and Partington 1998; Tager-Flusberg 1997). The selection of vocabulary words was based on a number of criteria, including meanings and intentions that are commonly expressed in early language communication and that can be practiced often. The specific criteria for vocabulary selection and target words/phrases for this study are presented in Table A.2. The thirty-six target words or two-word phrases were used in the pre- and post-tests. Both tests were in the same format, and were administered individually. The pre- and post-tests were a form of fill-in-the-blank, intraverbal communication.

In the present study, a music therapy technique called developmental speech and language training through music (DSLM) was used to address the acquisition of the target words/phrases. Six songs composed by me were used as music stimuli for the study. The songs included the thirty-six target words/phrases. Each song lyric included six target words/phrases, and each lyric line ended with a target word/phrase. Please see Appendix A for the complete notation of the songs. The same texts for the six songs used in the music stimuli were also used for the six stories in the speech stimuli.

Procedure

During the pre- and post-tests, data were collected in regard to each child's production of the target words/phrases. A correct verbal response consisted of four components: semantics, phonology, pragmatics, and prosody. These speech components tend to be most impaired in children with ASD (Rapin and Dunn 2003; Tager-Flusberg 2003). Some components such as pragmatics and prosody tend to be especially impaired in children with ASD (Rapin and Dunn 2003; Tager-Flusberg 2003). A verbal production evaluation scale designed by me measured participants' productions of the target words/phrases according to the four speech components (see Table A.3). One analysis of covariance (ANCOVA), a two-way analysis of variance (ANOVA), and an independent samples *t*-test were used to analyze the data.

Table A.2 Criteria for vocabulary word selection and target words/phrases

Criteria for vocabulary words	Target words/phrases	
Words that express early semantic functions		
Nonexistence or cessation	"all gone"	"all done"
Recurrence	"more"	"again"
Action	"stop"	"go"
Locative action	"down"	"out"
Words to request motivating things		
Food	"apple"	"banana"
Animals	"brown bear"	"pink pig"
Object	"key"	"shoe"
Words for routine independent living activities	"sing"	"story"
	"eat"	"sleep"
Words for expressing agreement of affirmation	"yes"	"okay"
Names (calling) of significant people	"mommy"	"baby"
Words to request		
Assistance	"help'	"here"
Affection or comfort	"kiss"	"hug"
Interaction	"play"	"come on"
Words for common environment	"home"	"school"
Action words of general application	"point"	"look"
Words of attribution	"pretty"	"dirty"
Words to express feelings or internal states	"happy"	"fun"

Table A.3 Verbal production evaluation scale

Instructions: Please answer each question by circling "Yes" or "No." Each item answered "Yes" is scored as 1 point. Participant Code: _____ Date: _____		
Target word/phrase:	Pre-test ( )	Post-test ( )
Semantics		
1. Does this verbal production include the correct target word/phrase?		
	Yes	No
Phonology		
2. Is the target word/phrase pronounced free of any articulation or phonetic errors?		
	Yes (free of error)	No (with error)
Pragmatics		
3. Is the target word/phrase produced at the right time, defined as ranging from immediate to within ten seconds?		
	Yes (produced in time)	No (not produced in time)
Prosody		
4. Is the target word/phrase produced with the proper pitch accent, given the context of the cue phrase?		
	Yes	No
5. Is the target word/phrase produced with the proper length of vowel sounds, given the context of the cue phrase?		
	Yes	No
6. Is the target word/phrase produced with the proper intensity (volume), given the context of the cue phrase?		
	Yes	No
	Total score: _____ points	

Results

Research question 1: Does level of speech production in children with ASD differ by training conditions: music versus speech versus no-training?

The effect of music and speech training on speech production in children with ASD

The results of this study showed that participants in both music and speech training increased their scores on the verbal production evaluation scale from the pre-test to the post-test. This finding suggests that both music and speech training are effective for enhancing speech production, including semantics, phonology, pragmatics, and prosody, in children with ASD. Participants who received music training gained a higher mean difference than participants who received the speech training; however, the difference was not statistically significant. In summary, music training is as effective as speech training for improving speech production.

The effect of music training on speech production in children with ASD

My observations suggest that participants in the music training responded to the target words/phrases and pictures more favorably than participants in the speech training. Participants in the music training maintained a seated position longer than participants in the speech training, and they showed fewer disruptive behaviors (e.g. shouting, crying, and tantrumming). Also, participants in the music training produced a higher number of target words/phrases. Some of the participants in the music training sang some lines in the songs and shouted target words/phrases during training sessions.

In addition, participants' anticipation for the beginnings and endings of the six songs during the music training was greater than the anticipation for the stories in the speech training. Some participants in the music training condition demonstrated a certain association for the songs by recalling the first phrase of each song. In summary, the music training seemed to draw more attention from the children with ASD than the speech training did. The children in the music training demonstrated more advanced cognitive skills from the increased attention such as anticipation, association, and recall of the stimuli during the training session and the post-test compared to children in the speech training.

Research question 2: Does level of speech production in children with ASD differ by level of functioning, language age, or presence of echolalia?

THE MAIN EFFECT OF LEVEL OF FUNCTIONING ON SPEECH PRODUCTION IN CHILDREN WITH ASD

The study showed that the previously determined level of functioning in the participants was a significant factor in target word/phrase production. The results revealed a significant difference between participants with a low level of functioning and a high level of functioning on speech production. High functioning children achieved higher scores on the post-test and a greater change from pre- to post-test scores on speech production than did low functioning children. The results also indicated that participants with a high level of functioning already knew many of the target words/phrases before the training, and improved target word/ phrase production after the music and speech training. Participants with a low level of functioning, however, did not score well on the pre-test, and scored much lower on the post-test than participants with a high level of functioning after the music and speech training. This finding suggests that a strong relationship exists between level of functioning and speech production in children with ASD. Speech production in children with ASD might be a critical factor to indicate their level of functioning.

THE INTERACTIVE EFFECT OF TRAINING CONDITION AND LEVEL OF FUNCTIONING

The study indicated a relationship between training conditions and participants' level of functioning for subsequent speech production. The results are presented in Figure A.1.

In summary, speech training might be an effective training tool to improve verbal production for children with a high level of functioning, but not for children with a low level of functioning. Music training might be an effective training tool to improve verbal production for children with either a high or a low level of functioning. In particular, children with a low level of functioning seem more likely to improve their speech production in response to music training.

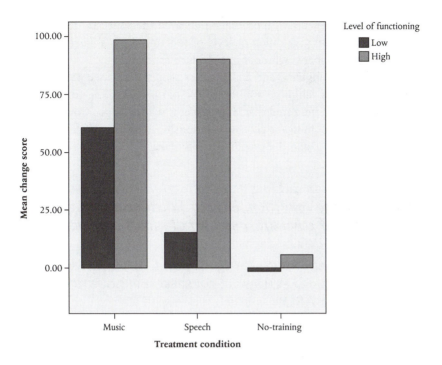

Figure A.1 The effects of training condition and level of functioning on verbal production

THE EFFECT OF ECHOLALIA AND LANGUAGE AGE ON SPEECH PRODUCTION

In my study, 64 percent of all participants showed echolalic behaviors. According to the results, the main effect of echolalia on participants' speech production was not statistically significant. The correlation coefficient analysis indicated that there was a significant relationship between echolalia and level of functioning in children with ASD, and that the two variables were positively related to each other. This finding suggests that children with ASD who produce echolalia are likely to also have a high level of functioning. Conversely, children with ASD who do not produce echolalia may have a low level of functioning. Logically, if echolalia is positively related to a high level of functioning, which is a critical factor for improved speech production, echolalia might be related to children's speech production as well. The results indicate that participants with echolalia achieved a much higher score on the post-test of speech production than participants who did not produce echolalia. In addition, participants with echolalia improved their speech production regardless of training condition or level of functioning to a much greater degree than participants who did not produce echolalia.

In the study, language age and pre-test scores were used to control the initial levels of language abilities in the participants. The correlation coefficient analysis indicated that language age, which ranged from one to four years, had a significant positive relationship with the pre-test score, level of functioning, and the presence of echolalia.

Research question 3: Does any interaction exist between type of training condition, level of functioning, language age, presence of echolalia, and overall speech production in children with ASD?

EFFECTS OF TRAINING CONDITIONS, LEVEL OF FUNCTIONING, LANGUAGE AGE, AND ECHOLALIA ON SPEECH PRODUCTION IN CHILDREN WITH ASD

The descriptive results of this study indicated that eight high functioning participants who received the music training achieved the highest mean score of all participants' groups on the post-test. Among the eight participants, seven participants produced echolalia, and one participant did not produce echolalia. Among ten low functioning participants who received the music training, six participants produced echolalia and four participants did not produce echolalia, and they achieved the lowest score in the music training condition. Among twelve high functioning participants who received the speech training, nine participants produced echolalia and three participants did not produce echolalia, and they achieved the highest score of all participants who received the speech training. Among six low functioning participants in the speech training condition, three participants produced echolalia and three participants did not produce echolalia. The children who were low functioning and did not produce echolalia achieved the lowest mean score of all participants in this study. All of the five high functioning participants in the no-training condition produced echolalia. Among the nine low functioning participants in the no-training condition, two participants produced echolalia and they achieved the lowest mean score of all participants, and seven participants did not produce echolalia.

The descriptive analysis indicated that, among all of the low functioning participants in this study (N = 25), six participants who produced echolalia and received the music training achieved the highest mean score. The analysis also indicated that three low functioning participants in the speech training who did not produce echolalia, and two low functioning participants in the no-training who produced echolalia, achieved the lowest mean score. The descriptive results indicated that, among all of the high functioning participants in this study (N = 25), 84 percent produced echolalia (N = 21). In contrast, among all of the low functioning participants (N = 25), only 44 percent of the participants produced echolalia (N = 11). The other 56 percent of the low functioning participants did not produce echolalia (N = 14). The presence of echolalia did not appear to interact with the training condition; however, it appeared to interact with level of functioning.

The inferential analysis indicated no significant interaction between training condition and the presence of echolalia after controlling for the pre-test score and language age, $F(2, 37) = 2.52$, $p = 0.94$. The analysis also indicated no significant interaction between training condition and level of functioning after controlling for the pre-test score and language age, $F(2, 37) = 0.65$, $p = 0.528$. Lastly, the results of the ANCOVA indicated no significant three-way interaction between training condition, echolalia, or level of functioning after controlling for the pre-test score and language age, $F(1, 37) = 0.41$, $p = 0.524$. The study therefore failed to reject the null hypothesis: there is no interaction between type of training condition, levels of functioning, language age, presence of echolalia, and speech production in children with ASD. All mean differences between the speech production in children with ASD are therefore explained by the main effects of the training condition and/or level of functioning.

RELATIONSHIPS AMONG LEVEL OF FUNCTIONING, ECHOLALIA, LANGUAGE AGE, AND THE PRE-TEST SCORE

The correlation analysis indicated that level of functioning, echolalia, language age, and the pre-test total score composite were positively correlated to each other and that the level of significance was considerably high. The most highly correlated variables were language age and level of functioning. The analysis showed that two covariates of language age and the pre-test total score also strongly correlated. Language age is also strongly correlated to echolalia. In addition, there was a strong correlation between the pre-test score and level of functioning, and between the pre-test score and echolalia.

According to the correlation analysis, the training condition did not appear to relate to any of the other independent variables or covariates. In fact, the training condition was an external variable, whereas other independent variables and covariates were internal variables acquired from the participants. The analysis indicated that the participants' language age was positively correlated to their level of functioning, which means that the high language age and high level of functioning were strongly related in the children with ASD ($r = 0.797$, $p = 0.000$). The analysis of correlation also indicated that the participants' language age was positively correlated to echolalia. High language age and the presence of echolalia were strongly related in the children with ASD ($r = 0.596$, $p = 0.000$). In addition, the result indicates that a high level of functioning and the presence of echolalia are strongly related in children with ASD ($r = 0.417$, $p = 0.003$).

Furthermore, the correlation analysis indicated that the participants' pre-test score was positively related to their language age ($r = 0.722$, $p = 0.000$), level of functioning ($r = 0.699$, $p = 0.000$), and the presence of echolalia ($r = 0.378$, $p = 0.007$). This particular result indicates that a participant's high score on the pre-test of the verbal production evaluation scale was strongly related to his or her high language age, high level of functioning, and the presence of echolalia.

Research question 4: Does any relationship exist between training conditions: music versus speech and various aspects of speech production, including semantics, phonology, pragmatics, and prosody, in children with ASD?

THE EFFECT OF TRAINING ON INDIVIDUAL COMPONENTS OF SPEECH PRODUCTION

The findings of this study indicate a significant effect of both music and speech training on speech production including semantics, phonology, pragmatics, and prosody in children with ASD. The results, however, revealed no significant difference between music and speech training on the four components of speech production: semantics, phonology, pragmatics, and prosody. In the study, both music and speech training improved all four components of speech production in just three days of training (i.e. six sessions).

According to the descriptive analysis, participants who received the music training improved three speech components—semantics, pragmatics, and prosody—to a greater degree than participants who received the speech training. Participants who received music training achieved a slightly higher score on the semantic component of the verbal production evaluation scale than participants who received speech training. This finding is congruent with the results indicating that a larger number of target words/phrases were produced by participants who received music training than speech training. For the other speech component, phonology, participants in both music and speech training achieved the same degree of improvement. Analysis of the raw data further revealed that two aspects of prosody, the volume (i.e. intensity) and the pitch accent, were increased to a greater degree from the pre-test to the post-test in participants who received music training compared to participants who received speech training. The other aspect of prosody, the length of vowel sounds, increased from the pre-test to the post-test to a similar degree by participants in both the music and speech training conditions.

Conclusion

This research suggests that developmental speech and language training through music is as effective as speech training for improving speech production in children with ASD. Presented music and speech stimuli were perceived as temporal patterns, and facilitated the verbal production of target words/phrases, including semantics, phonology, pragmatics, and prosody, in children with ASD through the repetition of training procedures. Music training resulted in greater improvement in speech production compared to speech training, in particular for low functioning children with ASD. The superior performance on speech production as well as enhanced attention in participants who received music training can be explained by the characteristics of the music stimuli. In this study, the music stimuli were composed using the Gestalt laws of pattern perception: the law of simplicity, similarity, proximity, common direction, and completion. However, the speech stimuli were developed using only the Gestalt principle of completion. The study suggests that children with ASD respond to music stimuli attentively and perceive important linguistic information (i.e. target words/phrases) embedded in the music stimuli. As a result, they can acquire and produce functional vocabulary words after receiving the developmental speech and language training through music. In conclusion, music is an effective tool for improving the acquisition of functional vocabulary words and speech production in children with ASD.

References

Adamek, M.S., Thaut, M.H. and Furman, A.G. (2008) "Individuals with Autism and Autism Spectrum Disorders." In D. Williams, K. Gfeller and M. Thaut (eds) *An Introduction to Music Therapy: Theory and Practice*, 3rd edn. Silver Spring, MD: American Music Therapy Association.

American Psychiatric Association (APA) (1994) *Diagnostic and Statistical Manual of Mental Disorders*, 4th edn. Washington, DC: APA.

Applebaum, E., Egel, A., Koegel, R. and Imhoff, B. (1979) "Measuring musical abilities of autistic children." *Journal of Autism and Developmental Disorders 9*, 279–285.

Barbera, M.L. (2007) *The Verbal Behavior Approach*. London: Jessica Kingsley Publishers.

Barrett, M. (1999) *The Development of Language*. Hove: Psychology Press.

Berger, D.S. (2002) *Music Therapy, Sensory Integration and the Autistic Child*. London: Jessica Kingsley Publishers.

Blackstock, E.G. (1978) "Cerebral asymmetry and the development of early infantile autism." *Journal of Autism and Childhood Schizophrenia 8*, 339–353.

Boddaert, N., Chabane, N., Belin, P., Bourgeois, M., *et al.* (2003) "Perception of complex sounds: Abnormal pattern of cortical activation in autism." *American Journal of Psychiatry 161*, 2057–2060.

Boddaert, N., Chabane, N., Belin, P., Bourgeois, M., *et al.* (2004) "Perception of complex sounds in autism: Abnormal auditory cortical processing in children." *American Journal of Psychiatry 161*, 2117–2120.

Bolinger, D. (1985) *Intonation and Its Parts: Melody in Spoken English*. London: Edward Arnold.

Boucher, J. (1988) "Word fluency in high-functioning autistic children." *Journal of Autism and Developmental Disorders 18*, 637–645.

Braithwaite, M. and Sigafoos, J. (1998) "Effects of social versus musical antecedents on communication responsiveness in five children with developmental disabilities." *Journal of Music Therapy 35*, 2, 88–104.

Brown, S., Martinez, M.J., Hodges, D.A., Fox, P.T. and Parsons, L.M. (2004) "The song system of the human brain." *Cognitive Brain Research 20*, 363–375.

Brown, S., Martinez, M.J. and Parsons, L.M. (2006) "Music and language side by side in the brain: A PET study of the generation of melodies and sentences." *European Journal of Neuroscience 23*, 2791–2803.

Brownell, M.D. (2002) "Musically adapted social stories to modify behaviors in students with autism: Four case studies." *Journal of Music Therapy 39*, 117–144.

Buday, E.M. (1995) "The effects of signed and spoken words taught with music on sign and speech imitation by children with autism." *Journal of Music Therapy 32*, 189–202.

Charman, T. and Baron-Cohen, S. (1994) "Another look at imitation in autism." *Development and Psychopathology 6*, 403–413.

Charman, T., Baron-Cohen, S., Swettenham, J., Baird, G., Drew, A. and Cox, A. (2003) "Predicting language outcome in infants with autism and pervasive developmental disorder." *International Journal of Language and Communication Disorders 38*, 265–285.

Chung, M.C., Jenner, L., Chamberlain, L. and Corbett, J. (1995) "One year follow-up pilot study on communication skill and challenging behavior." *European Journal of Psychiatry 9*, 83–95.

Clarke, E.F. (1987) "Categorical Rhythm Perception: An Ecological Perspective." In A. Gabrielsson (ed.) *Action and Perception in Rhythm in Music.* Stockholm: Royal Swedish Academy of Music.

Coleman, S. and Stedman, J. (1974) "Use of a peer model in language training in an echolalic child." *Journal of Behavioral Therapeutic Experiments in Psychiatry 5*, 275–279.

Delprato, D.J. (2001) "Comparison of discrete-trial and normalized behavioral language intervention for young children with autism." *Journal of Autism and Developmental Disorders 31*, 315–325.

Dunn, L.M. and Dunn, L.M. (1981) *Peabody Picture Vocabulary Test.* Circle Pines, MN: American Guidance Service.

Edgerton, C.L. (1994) "The effect of improvisational music therapy on the communicative behaviors of autistic children." *Journal of Music Therapy 31*, 31–62.

Eysenck, M.W. (2001) *Principles of Cognitive Psychology*, 2nd edn. Philadelphia, PA: Psychology Press.

Fay, W.H. (1969) "On the basis of autistic echolalia." *Journal of Communicative Disorders 2*, 38–47.

Fay, W.H. (1973) "On the echolalia of the blind and of the autistic child." *Journal of Speech and Hearing Disorders 38*, 478–489.

Frith, U. (1972) "Cognitive mechanisms in autism: Experiments with colors and tone sequence production." *Journal of Autism and Childhood Schizophrenia 2*, 160–173.

Frost, L. and Bondy, A. (1994) *The Picture Exchange Communication System Training Manual.* Cherry Hill, NJ: Pyramid Educational Consultants.

Gardner, M.F. (1979) *Expressive One-Word Picture Vocabulary Test.* Novato, CA: Academic Therapy Publications.

Goldstein, H. (2002) "Communication intervention for children with autism: A review of treatment efficacy." *Journal of Autism and Developmental Disorders 32*, 373–396.

Green, G., Brennan, L.C. and Fein, D. (2002) "Intensive behavioral treatment for a toddler at high risk for autism." *Behavior Modification 26*, 69–102.

Hafteck, L. (1997) "Music and language development in early childhood: Integrating past research in the two domains." *Early Child Development and Care 130*, 85–97.

Heaton, P., Hermelin, B. and Pring, L. (1999) "Can children with autistic spectrum disorder perceive affect in music? An experimental investigation." *Psychological Medicine 29*, 1405–1410.

Hoskins, C. (1988) "Use of music to increase verbal response and improve expressive language abilities of preschool language delayed children." *Journal of Music Therapy 25*, 73–84.

Jones, E., Feeley, K. and Takacs, J. (2007) "Teaching spontaneous responses to young children with autism." *Journal of Applied Behavior Analysis 40*, 565–570.

Kanner, L. (1946) "Irrelevant and metaphorical language in early infantile autism." *American Journal of Psychiatry 103*, 242–246.

Kaplan, R.S. and Steele, A.L. (2005) "An analysis of music therapy program goals and outcomes for clients with diagnoses on the autism spectrum." *Journal of Music Therapy 42*, 2–19.

Koegel, L.K. (2000) "Interventions to facilitate communication in autism." *Journal of Autism and Developmental Disorders 30*, 383–391.

Koegel, R.L., Lovaas, I. and Schreibman, L. (1974) "A behavioral modification approach to the treatment of autistic children." *Journal of Autism and Developmental Disorders 4*, 111–129.

Kolko, D.J., Anderson, L. and Campbell, M. (1980) "Sensory preference and overselective responding in autistic children." *Journal of Autism and Developmental Disorders 10*, 259–271.

Kostka, S. and Payne, D. (2000) *Tonal Harmony*. Boston: McGraw Hill.

Krashen, S. and Scarcella, R. (1978) "On routines and patterns in language acquisition and performance." *Language Learning 28*, 283–300.

Lim, H.A. (2009) "Use of music to improve speech production in children with autism spectrum disorders: Theoretical orientation." *Music Therapy Perspectives 27*, 2, 103–114.

Lim, H.A. (2010) "The effect of "developmental speech-language training through music" on speech production in children with autism spectrum disorders." *Journal of Music Therapy 47*, 1, 2–26.

Lipscomb, S.D. (1996) "The Cognitive Organization of Musical Sound." In D.A. Hodges (ed.) *Handbook of Music Psychology*, 2nd edn. San Antonio, TX: IMR Press.

Lord, C. and Paul, R. (1997) "Language and Communication in Autism." In D. Cohen and F. Volkmar (eds) *Handbook of Autism and Pervasive Developmental Disorders*. New York: Wiley.

Lovaas, O.I. (1977) *The Autistic Child: Language Development through Behavior Modification*. New York: Irvington.

McCann, J. and Peppe, S. (2003) "Prosody in autism spectrum disorders: A critical review." *International Journal of Language and Communication Disorders 38*, 4, 325–350.

McMullen, E. and Saffran, J.R. (2004) "Music and language: A developmental comparison." *Music Perception 21*, 289–311.

Mancil, R., Conroy, M. and Haydon, T. (2009) "Effects of a modified milieu therapy intervention on the social communicative behaviors of young children with autism spectrum disorders." *Journal of Autism and Developmental Disorders 39*, 149–163.

Maurice, C., Green, G. and Luce, S.C. (eds) (1996) *Behavior Intervention for Young Children with Autism.* Austin, TX: Pro-Ed.

Michel, D.E. and Jones, J.L. (1992) *Music for Developing Speech and Language Skills in Children: A Guide for Parents and Therapists.* St Louis, MO: MMB Music.

Minshew, N.J. and Goldstein, G. (1993) "Is autism an amnesic disorder? Evidence from the California Verbal Learning Test." *Neuropsychology 7*, 209–216.

National Research Council (NRC) (Committee on Educational Interventions for Children with Autism, Division of Behavioral and Social Sciences and Education) (2001) *Educating Children with Autism.* Washington, DC: National Academy Press.

Nelson, D.I., Anderson, V.G. and Gonzales, A.D. (1984) "Music activities as therapy for children with autism and other pervasive developmental disorders." *Journal of Music Therapy 21*, 100–116.

O'Connell, T. (1974) "The musical life of an autistic boy." *Journal of Autism and Childhood Schizophrenia 4*, 223–229.

Orr, T.J., Myles, B.S. and Carlson, J.K. (1998) "The impact of rhythmic entrainment on a person with autism." *Focus on Autism and Other Developmental Disabilities 13*, 163–166.

Patel, A.D. (2003) "Language, music, syntax and the brain." *Nature Neuroscience 6*, 674–681.

Patel, A.D. (2008) *Music, Language and the Brain.* Oxford: Oxford University Press.

Patel, A.D., Peretz, I., Tramo, M. and Labreque, R. (1998) "Processing prosodic and musical patterns: A neuropsychological investigation." *Brain and Language 61*, 123–144.

Paul, R. and Sutherland, D. (2005) "Enhancing Early Language in Children with Autism Spectrum Disorders." In F. Volkmar, R. Paul, A. Ktin and D. Cohen (eds) *Handbook of Autism and Pervasive Developmental Disorders.* New York: Wiley.

Peretz, I., Gagnon, L., Hebert, S. and Macoir, J. (2004) "Singing in the brain: Insights from cognitive neuropsychology." *Music Perception 21*, 373–390.

Peters, A.M. (1977) "Language learning strategies: Does the whole equal the sum of the part?" *Language 53*, 560–573.

Peters, A.M. (1980) "The units of language acquisition." *Working Papers in Linguistics 12*, 1–72.

Peters, A.M. (1983) *The Units of Language Acquisition.* London: Cambridge University Press.

Price, C.J., Wise, R.J., Warburton, E.A., Moore, C.J., *et al.* (1996) "Hearing and saying: The functional neuro-anatomy of auditory word processing." *Brain 119*, 919–931.

Prizant, B.M. (1983) "Language acquisition and communicative behavior in autism: Toward an understanding of the "whole" of it." *Journal of Speech and Hearing Disorders 48*, 296–307.

Prizant, B.M. (1987) "Clinical Implications of Echolalic Behavior in Autism." In T. Layton (ed.) *Language and Treatment of Autistic and Developmentally Disordered Children.* Springfield, IL: Charles C. Thomas.

Prizant, B.M. and Duchan, J.F. (1981) "The functions of immediate echolalia in autistic children." *Journal of Speech and Hearing Disorders 46*, 241–249.

Prizant, B.M. and Wetherby, A.M. (1993) "Communication in Preschool Autistic Children." In E. Schopler, M. Van Bourgandien and M. Bristol (eds) *Preschool Issues in Autism*. New York: Plenum Press.

Prizant, B.M. and Wetherby, A.M. (2005) "Critical Issues in Enhancing Communication Abilities for Persons with Autism Spectrum Disorders." In F. Volkmar, R. Paul, A. Ktin and D. Cohen (eds) *Handbook of Autism and Pervasive Developmental Disorders*. New York: Wiley.

Prizant, B.M., Schuler, A.L., Wetherby, A.M. and Rydell, P. (1997) "Enhancing Language and Communication Development: Language Approaches." In D. Cohen and F. Volkmar (eds) *Handbook of Autism and Pervasive Developmental Disorders*. New York: Wiley.

Radocy, R.E. and Boyle, J.D. (2003) *Psychological Foundation of Musical Behavior*, 4th edn. Springfield, IL: Charles C. Thomas.

Rapin, I. and Dunn, M. (2003) "Update of the language disorders of individuals on the autistic spectrum." *Brain and Development 25*, 166–172.

Roberts, T.P., Schmidt, H.C., Egeth, M., Blaskey, L., Rey, M., Edgar, J.C. and Levy, S. (2008) "Electrophysiological signatures: Magnetoencephalographic studies of the neural correlates of language impairment in autism spectrum disorders." *International Journal of Psychophysiology 10*, 1016, 1–12.

Rydell, P.J. and Mirenda, P. (1991) "The effects of two levels of linguistic constraint on echolalia and generative language production in children with autism." *Journal of Autism and Developmental Disorders 21*, 131–158.

Rydell, P.J. and Prizant, B.M. (1995) "Assessment and Intervention Strategies for Children Who Use Echolalia." In K. Quill (ed.) *Teaching Children with Autism*. New York: Delmar.

Scherer, N. and Olswang, L. (1989) "Using structured discourse as a language intervention technique with autistic children." *Journal of Speech and Hearing Disorders 54*, 383–394.

Schön, D., Magne, C. and Besson, M. (2004) "The music of speech: Music training facilitates pitch processing in both music and language." *Psychophysiology 41*, 341–349.

Schreibman, L. and Carr, E. (1978) "Elimination of echolalic responding to questions through the training of a generalized verbal response." *Journal of Applied Behavioral Analysis 11*, 453–464.

Schuler, A.L. (1995) "Thinking in Autism: Differences in Learning and Development." In K. Quill (ed.) *Teaching Children with Autism: Methods to Enhance Communication and Socialization*. Albany, NY: Delmar.

Seybold, C.D. (1971) "The value and use of music activities in the treatment of speech delayed children." *Journal of Music Therapy 8*, 102–110.

Shafer, E. (1994) "A review of interventions to teach a mand repertoire." *Analysis of Verbal Behavior 12*, 53–66.

Sherwin, A. (1953) "Reactions to music of autistic children." *American Journal of Psychiatry 109*, 823–831.

Sigafoos, J. (2000) "Communication development and aberrant behavior in children with developmental disabilities." *Education and Training in Mental Retardation and Developmental Disabilities 35*, 168–176.

Skinner, B.F. (1957) *Verbal Behavior*. Englewood Cliffs, NJ: Prentice Hall.

Sloboda, J.A. (1985) *The Musical Mind*. Oxford: Clarendon Press.

Stevens, E. and Clark, F. (1969) "Music therapy in the treatment of autistic children." *Journal of Music Therapy 6*, 98–104.

Sturmey, P. and Fitzer, A. (2007) *Autism Spectrum Disorders: Applied Behavior Analysis, Evidence, and Practice*. Austin, TX: Pro-Ed.

Sundberg, M.L. and Michael, J. (2001) "The benefits of Skinner's analysis of verbal behavior for children with autism." *Behavior Modification 25*, 698–724.

Sundberg, M.L. and Partington, J.W. (1998) *Teaching Language to Children with Autism or Other Developmental Disabilities*. Pleasant Hill, CA: Behavior Analysts.

Sundberg, M.L., Loeb, M., Hale, L. and Eigenheer, P. (2002) "Contriving establishing operations to teach mands for information." *The Analysis of Verbal Behavior 18*, 15–29.

Sundberg, M.L., Michael, J. and Partington, J.W. (1996) "The role of automatic reinforcement in early language acquisition." *Analysis of Verbal Behavior 12*, 21–37.

Tager-Flusberg, H. (1981) "On the nature of linguistic functioning in early infantile autism." *Journal of Autism and Developmental Disorders 1*, 45–56.

Tager-Flusberg, H. (1985) "The conceptual basis for referential word meaning in children with autism." *Child Development 56*, 1167–1178.

Tager-Flusberg, H. (1986) "Constraints on the Representation of Word Meaning: Evidence from Autistic and Mentally Retarded Children." In S.A. Kuczaj and M. Barrett (eds) *The Development of Word Meaning*. New York: Springer.

Tager-Flusberg, H. (1991) "Semantic processing in the free recall of autistic children: Further evidence for a cognitive deficit." *British Journal of Developmental Psychology 9*, 417–430.

Tager-Flusberg, H. (1997) "Perspectives on Language and Communication in Autism." In D. Cohen and F. Volkmar (eds) *Handbook of Autism and Pervasive Developmental Disorders*. New York: Wiley.

Tager-Flusberg, H. (2003) "Language Impairment in Children with Complex Neurodevelopmental Disorders: The Case of Autism." In Y. Levy and J. Schaeffer (eds) *Language Competence across Population: Toward a Definition of Specific Language Impairment*. Mahwah, NJ: Lawrence Erlbaum.

Tager-Flusberg, H. and Calkins, S. (1990) "Does imitation facilitate the acquisition of grammar? Evidence from a study of autistic, Down syndrome and normal children." *Journal of Child Language 17*, 591–606.

Tager-Flusberg, H., Calkins, S., Nolin, T., Baumberger, T., Anderson, M. and Chadwick-Dias, A. (1990) "A longitudinal study of language acquisition in autistic and Down syndrome children." *Journal of Autism and Developmental Disorders 20*, 1–21.

Thaut, M.H. (1987) "Visual vs. auditory (musical) stimulus preferences in autistic children." *Journal of Autism and Developmental Disorders 17*, 425–432.

Thaut, M.H. (1988) "Measuring musical responsiveness in autistic children: A comparative analysis of improvised musical tone sequences of autistic, normal and mentally retarded individuals." *Journal of Autism and Developmental Disorders 18*, 561–571.

Thaut, M.H. (1999) "Music Therapy with Autistic Children." In W. Davis, K. Gfeller and M. Thaut (eds) *An Introduction to Music Therapy: Theory and Practice*, 2nd edn. Boston, MA: McGraw-Hill.

Thaut, M.H. (2005) *Rhythm, Music, and the Brain: Scientific Foundations and Clinical Applications.* New York: Routledge.

Travis, L. and Sigman, M. (2001) "Links between social understanding and social behavior in verbally able children with autism." *Journal of Autism and Developmental Disorders 31*, 119–130.

Trehub, S.E. and Trainor, L.J. (1993) "Listening Strategies in Infancy: The Roots of Music and Language Development." In S. McAdams and E. Bigand (eds) *Thinking in Sound: The Cognitive Psychology of Hearing and Audition.* Oxford: Oxford University Press.

Volden, J. and Lord, C. (1991) "Neologisms and idiosyncratic language in autistic speakers." *Journal of Autism and Developmental Disorders 21*, 109–130.

Walker, J.B. (1972) "The use of music as an aid in developing functional speech in the institutionalized mentally retarded." *Journal of Music Therapy 9*, 1–12.

Wetherby, A.M. and Woods, J. (2008) "Developmental Approaches to Treatment." In K. Chawarskia, A. Klin and F.R. Volkmar (eds) *Autism Spectrum Disorders in Infants and Toddlers.* New York: Guilford Press.

Whipple, J. (2004) "Music in intervention for children and adolescents with autism: A meta-analysis." *Journal of Music Therapy 41*, 90–106.

Wigram, T. (2000) "A method of music therapy assessment for the diagnosis of autism and communication disorders in children." *Music Therapy Perspectives 18*, 13–18.

Wimpory, D. and Nash, S. (1999) "Musical interaction therapy: Therapeutic play for children with autism." *Child Language Teaching and Therapy 15*, 17–28.

Wise, R.J., Scott, S.K., Blank, S.C., Mummery, C.J., Murphy, K. and Warburton, E.A. (2001) "Separate neural subsystems within 'Wernicke's area'." *Brain 124*, 83–95.

Subject Index

Author Index